# 2. Filet mignon

## Ingredient:

• 2 filet mignon steaks, about 6•8 oz each
• Salt and pepper to taste

## Instructions:

1. Pat the filet mignon steaks dry with paper towels and season generously with salt and pepper on all sides.

2. Heat a cast•iron skillet or heavy•bottomed pan over high heat. Once the pan is very hot, add the steaks and sear for 2•3 minutes per side, or until a nice brown crust forms.

3. Reduce the heat to medium•low and continue cooking the steaks, flipping occasionally, until they reach your desired doneness. For medium•rare, this will take about 8•10 minutes total.

4. Transfer the steaks to a cutting board and let them rest for 5•10 minutes before slicing and serving.

Tips:
• Choose high•quality, fresh filet mignon for the best flavor and tenderness.

• Avoid overcooking the steaks, as filet mignon can become dry and tough if cooked past medium•rare.

• Serve the steaks with no additional sides or sauces to keep it true to the carnivore diet.

• Drink plenty of water and stay hydrated when following a carnivore diet.

# 3. Sirloin steak

## Ingredient:

• 2 sirloin steaks, about 6•8 oz each
• Salt and pepper to taste

## Instructions:

1. Pat the sirloin steaks dry with paper towels and season generously with salt and pepper on all sides.

2. Heat a cast•iron skillet or heavy•bottomed pan over high heat. Once the pan is very hot, add the steaks and sear for 2•3 minutes per side, or until a nice brown crust forms.

3. Reduce the heat to medium•low and continue cooking the steaks, flipping occasionally, until they reach your desired doneness. For medium•rare, this will take about 8•10 minutes total.

4. Transfer the steaks to a cutting board and let them rest for 5•10 minutes before slicing and serving.

Tips:
• Choose a high•quality, well•marbled sirloin for maximum flavor and tenderness.

• Avoid overcooking the steaks, as sirloin can become tough if cooked past medium•rare.

• Serve the steaks with no additional sides or sauces to keep it true to the carnivore diet.

• Drink plenty of water and stay hydrated when following a carnivore diet.

Welcome to ***100+ Recipes Carnivore Diet Cookbook for Men: Fuel Your Strength and Vitality with Delicious Meat-Based Recipes.*** This cookbook is your essential companion on the journey to embracing the carnivore diet—a dietary approach that focuses exclusively on animal products—to enhance your strength, vitality, and overall well-being.

## Embracing the Carnivore Diet

The carnivore diet has gained popularity for its potential benefits such as reduced inflammation, improved digestion, stable energy levels, and enhanced mental clarity. For men, this dietary approach offers the opportunity to fuel your body with nutrient-dense, protein-rich foods that support muscle growth, recovery, and sustained energy throughout the day.

## What You'll Discover in This Book

*Inside these pages, you'll find:*

- ***100+ Delicious Recipes:*** From hearty breakfasts and satisfying lunches to flavorful dinners and indulgent desserts, each recipe is crafted to maximize flavor and nutrition using a variety of meat, poultry, fish, and other animal products.

- ***Simple and Practical Cooking:*** We understand the demands of modern life, so the recipes are designed to be straightforward and easy to follow. Whether you're a novice or an experienced cook, you'll find these dishes accessible and enjoyable to prepare.

- ***Nutritional Benefits:*** Explore the nutritional benefits of the carnivore diet for men, including how it can support muscle maintenance, hormone balance, and overall physical performance.

- ***Holistic Health Tips:*** Beyond recipes, this book offers insights into lifestyle practices such as exercise, hydration, and stress management that complement your dietary choices and contribute to your overall health and vitality.

## Empowerment Through Nutrition

By choosing to explore the carnivore diet, you're making a commitment to prioritize your health and optimize your performance. This cookbook aims to empower you with the knowledge and tools needed to succeed on your carnivore journey, while enjoying delicious and satisfying meals that fuel your strength and vitality.

**A Note on Your Journey**

Whether you're new to the carnivore diet or looking to refine your approach, this book is here to support you. Embrace the adventure of discovering new flavors, nourishing your body with high-quality ingredients, and experiencing the benefits of a diet tailored specifically for men's health.

*Thank you for embarking on this journey with us. Here's to delicious meals, renewed energy, and a vibrant, healthy life fueled by the carnivore diet.*

# 1. Ribeye steak

## Ingredient:

• 1 ribeye steak, about 8•10 oz
• Salt and pepper to taste

## Instructions:

1. Pat the ribeye steak dry with paper towels and season generously with salt and pepper on both sides.

2. Heat a cast•iron skillet or heavy•bottomed pan over high heat. Once the pan is very hot, add the steak and sear for 2•3 minutes per side, or until a nice brown crust forms.

3. Reduce the heat to medium•low and continue cooking the steak, flipping occasionally, until it reaches your desired doneness. For medium•rare, this will take about 5•7 minutes total.

4. Transfer the steak to a cutting board and let it rest for 5•10 minutes before slicing and serving.

Tips:
• Choose a high•quality, well•marbled ribeye for maximum flavor and tenderness.

• Avoid overcooking the steak, as this can make it tough. Aim for medium•rare to medium doneness.

• Serve the steak with no additional sides or sauces to keep it true to the carnivore diet.

• Drink plenty of water and stay hydrated when following a carnivore diet.

# 4. New York strip steak

## Ingredient:

• 2 New York strip steaks, about 8•10 oz each
• Salt and pepper to taste

## Instructions:

1. Pat the New York strip steaks dry with paper towels and season generously with salt and pepper on all sides.

2. Heat a cast•iron skillet or heavy•bottomed pan over high heat. Once the pan is very hot, add the steaks and sear for 2•3 minutes per side, or until a nice brown crust forms.

3. Reduce the heat to medium•low and continue cooking the steaks, flipping occasionally, until they reach your desired doneness. For medium•rare, this will take about 8•10 minutes total.

4. Transfer the steaks to a cutting board and let them rest for 5•10 minutes before slicing and serving.

Tips:
• Choose a high•quality, well•marbled New York strip for maximum flavor and tenderness.
• Avoid overcooking the steaks, as New York strip can become tough if cooked past medium•rare.
• Serve the steaks with no additional sides or sauces to keep it true to the carnivore diet.
• Drink plenty of water and stay hydrated when following a carnivore diet.

# 5. Lamb chops

**Ingredient:**

• 4 lamb chops, about 4•6 oz each
• Salt and pepper to taste

**Instructions**:

1. Pat the lamb chops dry with paper towels and season generously with salt and pepper on both sides.

2. Heat a cast•iron skillet or heavy•bottomed pan over high heat. Once the pan is very hot, add the lamb chops and sear for 2•3 minutes per side, or until a nice brown crust forms.

3. Reduce the heat to medium•low and continue cooking the lamb chops, flipping occasionally, until they reach your desired doneness. For medium•rare, this will take about 8•10 minutes total.

4. Transfer the lamb chops to a cutting board and let them rest for 5•10 minutes before serving.

Tips:
• Choose high•quality, pasture•raised lamb chops for the best flavor and tenderness.

• Avoid overcooking the lamb chops, as they can become tough if cooked past medium•rare.

• Serve the lamb chops with no additional sides or sauces to keep it true to the carnivore diet.

• Drink plenty of water and stay hydrated when following a carnivore diet.

# 6. Pork chops

## Ingredient:

• 4 bone•in pork chops, about 6•8 oz each
• Salt and pepper to taste

## Instructions:

1. Pat the pork chops dry with paper towels and season generously with salt and pepper on both sides.

2. Heat a cast•iron skillet or heavy•bottomed pan over high heat. Once the pan is very hot, add the pork chops and sear for 2•3 minutes per side, or until a nice brown crust forms.

3. Reduce the heat to medium•low and continue cooking the pork chops, flipping occasionally, until they reach an internal temperature of 145°F. This will take about 8•10 minutes total.

4. Transfer the pork chops to a cutting board and let them rest for 5•10 minutes before serving.

Tips:
• Choose bone•in pork chops for maximum flavor and tenderness.

• Avoid overcooking the pork chops, as they can become dry and tough if cooked past 145°F.

• Serve the pork chops with no additional sides or sauces to keep it true to the carnivore diet.

• Drink plenty of water and stay hydrated when following a carnivore diet.

# 7. Ground beef patties

## Ingredient:

• 1 lb ground beef (preferably 80/20 or 85/15 blend)
• Salt and pepper to taste

## Instructions:

1. Divide the ground beef into 4 equal portions and gently shape them into patties, being careful not to overwork the meat.

2. Season the patties generously with salt and pepper on both sides.

3. Heat a cast•iron skillet or heavy•bottomed pan over high heat. Once the pan is very hot, add the patties and sear for 2•3 minutes per side, or until a nice brown crust forms.

4. Reduce the heat to medium•low and continue cooking the patties, flipping occasionally, until they reach your desired doneness. For medium•rare, this will take about 5•7 minutes total.

5. Transfer the patties to a plate and let them rest for 5 minutes before serving.

Tips:
• Use a high•quality, freshly ground beef for the best flavor and texture.

• Avoid overworking the meat when shaping the patties, as this can make them tough.

• Adjust the cooking time based on your preferred level of doneness, but be careful not to overcook the patties.

• Serve the patties with no additional sides or sauces to keep it true to the carnivore diet.

• Drink plenty of water and stay hydrated when following a carnivore diet.

# 8. Beef tenderloin

**Ingredient:**

• 1 beef tenderloin, about 2•3 lbs
• Salt and pepper to taste

**Instructions**:

1. Pat the beef tenderloin dry with paper towels and season generously with salt and pepper all over.

2. Preheat your oven to 400°F (200°C).

3. Heat a large, oven•safe skillet or cast•iron pan over high heat. Once the pan is very hot, sear the tenderloin on all sides until a nice brown crust forms, about 2•3 minutes per side.

4. Transfer the pan to the preheated oven and roast the tenderloin until it reaches your desired level of doneness. For medium•rare, this will take about 20•25 minutes.

5. Remove the tenderloin from the oven and let it rest for 10•15 minutes before slicing and serving.

Tips:
• Choose a high•quality, center•cut beef tenderloin for the best texture and flavor.

• Be careful not to overcook the tenderloin, as it can become dry and tough if cooked past medium•rare.

• Serve the tenderloin slices with no additional sides or sauces to keep it true to the carnivore diet.

• Drink plenty of water and stay hydrated when following a carnivore diet.

# 9. Venison steak

## Ingredient:

• 2 venison steaks, about 6•8 oz each
• Salt and pepper to taste

## Instructions:

1. Pat the venison steaks dry with paper towels and season generously with salt and pepper on both sides.

2. Heat a cast•iron skillet or heavy•bottomed pan over high heat. Once the pan is very hot, add the venison steaks and sear for 2•3 minutes per side, or until a nice brown crust forms.

3. Reduce the heat to medium•low and continue cooking the steaks, flipping occasionally, until they reach your desired doneness. For medium•rare, this will take about 6•8 minutes total.

4. Transfer the steaks to a cutting board and let them rest for 5•10 minutes before slicing and serving.

Tips:
• Choose high•quality, fresh venison for the best flavor and tenderness.

• Venison is a lean meat, so be careful not to overcook it, as it can become tough and dry.

• Serve the venison steaks with no additional sides or sauces to keep it true to the carnivore diet.

• Drink plenty of water and stay hydrated when following a carnivore diet.

# 10. Bison burger

## Ingredient:

• 1 lb ground bison
• Salt and pepper to taste

## Instructions:

1. Divide the ground bison into 4 equal portions and gently shape them into patties, being careful not to overwork the meat.

2. Season the patties generously with salt and pepper on both sides.

3. Heat a cast•iron skillet or heavy•bottomed pan over high heat. Once the pan is very hot, add the bison patties and sear for 2•3 minutes per side, or until a nice brown crust forms.

4. Reduce the heat to medium•low and continue cooking the patties, flipping occasionally, until they reach your desired doneness. For medium•rare, this will take about 5•7 minutes total.

5. Transfer the patties to a plate and let them rest for 5 minutes before serving.

Tips:
• Use high•quality, freshly ground bison for the best flavor and texture.

• Avoid overworking the meat when shaping the patties, as this can make them tough.

• Adjust the cooking time based on your preferred level of doneness, but be careful not to overcook the patties.

• Serve the bison burgers with no additional sides or sauces to keep it true to the carnivore diet.

• Drink plenty of water and stay hydrated when following a carnivore diet.

# 11. Veal cutlets

## Ingredient:

• 4 veal cutlets, about 4•6 oz each
• Salt and pepper to taste

## Instructions:

1. Pat the veal cutlets dry with paper towels and season generously with salt and pepper on both sides.

2. Heat a cast•iron skillet or heavy•bottomed pan over high heat. Once the pan is very hot, add the veal cutlets and sear for 2•3 minutes per side, or until a nice brown crust forms.

3. Reduce the heat to medium•low and continue cooking the cutlets, flipping occasionally, until they reach your desired doneness. For medium•rare, this will take about 5•7 minutes total.

4. Transfer the veal cutlets to a plate and let them rest for 5 minutes before serving.

Tips:
• Choose high•quality, fresh veal cutlets for the best flavor and tenderness.

• Avoid overcooking the veal, as it can become tough and dry if cooked past medium•rare.

• Serve the veal cutlets with no additional sides or sauces to keep it true to the carnivore diet.

• Drink plenty of water and stay hydrated when following a carnivore diet.

# 12. Chicken thighs

## Ingredient:

• 4 bone•in, skin•on chicken thighs
• Salt and pepper to taste

## Instructions:

1. Pat the chicken thighs dry with paper towels and season generously with salt and pepper on both sides.

2. Heat a cast•iron skillet or heavy•bottomed pan over medium•high heat. Once the pan is hot, add the chicken thighs, skin•side down, and sear for 5•7 minutes, or until the skin is crispy and golden brown.

3. Flip the chicken thighs and continue cooking for another 5•7 minutes, or until the internal temperature reaches 165°F.

4. Transfer the chicken thighs to a plate and let them rest for 5 minutes before serving.

Tips:
• Choose bone•in, skin•on chicken thighs for maximum flavor and juiciness.

• Avoid overcooking the chicken, as it can become dry and tough if cooked past 165°F.

• Serve the chicken thighs with no additional sides or sauces to keep it true to the carnivore diet.

• Drink plenty of water and stay hydrated when following a carnivore diet.

# 13. Chicken drumsticks

## Ingredient:

• 6 chicken drumsticks
• Salt and pepper to taste

## Instructions:

1. Pat the chicken drumsticks dry with paper towels and season generously with salt and pepper on all sides.

2. Heat a cast•iron skillet or heavy•bottomed pan over medium•high heat. Once the pan is hot, add the chicken drumsticks and sear for 5•7 minutes per side, or until the skin is crispy and golden brown.

3. Reduce the heat to medium•low and continue cooking the drumsticks, turning occasionally, until the internal temperature reaches 165°F, about 15•20 minutes total.

4. Transfer the chicken drumsticks to a plate and let them rest for 5 minutes before serving.

Tips:
• Choose fresh, high•quality chicken drumsticks for the best flavor and texture.

• Avoid overcooking the drumsticks, as they can become dry and tough if cooked past 165°F.

• Serve the chicken drumsticks with no additional sides or sauces to keep it true to the carnivore diet.

• Drink plenty of water and stay hydrated when following a carnivore diet.

# 14. Chicken wings

## Ingredient:

• 12 chicken wings, drumettes and flats separated
• Salt and pepper to taste

## Instructions:

1. Pat the chicken wings dry with paper towels and season generously with salt and pepper on all sides.

2. Heat a cast•iron skillet or heavy•bottomed pan over medium•high heat. Once the pan is hot, add the chicken wings in a single layer and sear for 5•7 minutes per side, or until the skin is crispy and golden brown.

3. Reduce the heat to medium•low and continue cooking the wings, turning occasionally, until the internal temperature reaches 165°F, about 15•20 minutes total.

4. Transfer the chicken wings to a plate and let them rest for 5 minutes before serving.

Tips:
• Choose fresh, high•quality chicken wings for the best flavor and texture.

• Avoid overcooking the wings, as they can become dry and tough if cooked past 165°F.

• Serve the chicken wings with no additional sides or sauces to keep it true to the carnivore diet.

• Drink plenty of water and stay hydrated when following a carnivore diet.

# 15. Duck breast

## Ingredient:

• 2 duck breasts, about 6•8 oz each
• Salt and pepper to taste

## Instructions:

1. Pat the duck breasts dry with paper towels and season generously with salt and pepper on both sides.

2. Heat a cast•iron skillet or heavy•bottomed pan over medium•high heat. Once the pan is hot, add the duck breasts, skin•side down, and sear for 5•7 minutes, or until the skin is crispy and golden brown.

3. Flip the duck breasts and continue cooking for another 5•7 minutes, or until the internal temperature reaches 130°F for medium•rare.

4. Transfer the duck breasts to a cutting board and let them rest for 5•10 minutes before slicing and serving.

Tips:
• Choose high•quality, fresh duck breasts for the best flavor and texture.

• Be careful not to overcook the duck, as it can become tough and dry if cooked past medium•rare.

• Serve the sliced duck breast with no additional sides or sauces to keep it true to the carnivore diet.

• Drink plenty of water and stay hydrated when following a carnivore diet.

# 16. Turkey legs

## Ingredient:

- 2 turkey legs
- Salt and pepper to taste

## Instructions:

1. Pat the turkey legs dry with paper towels and season generously with salt and pepper on all sides.

2. Preheat your oven to 375°F (190°C).

3. Place the seasoned turkey legs in a roasting pan or baking dish. Roast for 60•75 minutes, or until the internal temperature reaches 165°F.

4. Remove the turkey legs from the oven and let them rest for 10•15 minutes before serving.

Tips:
- Choose fresh, high•quality turkey legs for the best flavor and texture.

- Avoid overcooking the turkey legs, as they can become dry and tough if cooked past 165°F.

- Serve the turkey legs with no additional sides or sauces to keep it true to the carnivore diet.

- Drink plenty of water and stay hydrated when following a carnivore diet.

# 17. Quail

**Ingredient:**

• 4 quail, whole
• Salt and pepper to taste

**Instructions**:

1. Pat the quail dry with paper towels and season generously with salt and pepper on all sides.

2. Heat a cast•iron skillet or heavy•bottomed pan over medium•high heat. Once the pan is hot, add the quail, breast•side down, and sear for 3•4 minutes, or until the skin is crispy and golden brown.

3. Flip the quail and continue cooking for another 3•4 minutes.

4. Transfer the pan to a preheated 400°F (200°C) oven and roast the quail for an additional 10•12 minutes, or until the internal temperature reaches 165°F.

5. Remove the quail from the oven and let them rest for 5 minutes before serving.

Tips:
• Choose fresh, high•quality quail for the best flavor and tenderness.

• Avoid overcooking the quail, as they can become dry and tough if cooked past 165°F.

• Serve the quail with no additional sides or sauces to keep it true to the carnivore diet.

• Drink plenty of water and stay hydrated when following a carnivore diet.

# 18. Goose breast

## Ingredient:

• 2 goose breasts, about 8•10 oz each
• Salt and pepper to taste

## Instructions:

1. Pat the goose breasts dry with paper towels and season generously with salt and pepper on both sides.

2. Heat a cast•iron skillet or heavy•bottomed pan over medium•high heat. Once the pan is hot, add the goose breasts, skin•side down, and sear for 7•10 minutes, or until the skin is crispy and golden brown.

3. Flip the goose breasts and continue cooking for another 5•7 minutes, or until the internal temperature reaches 130°F for medium•rare.

4. Transfer the goose breasts to a cutting board and let them rest for 10 minutes before slicing and serving.

Tips:
• Choose high•quality, fresh goose breasts for the best flavor and texture.

• Be careful not to overcook the goose, as it can become tough and dry if cooked past medium•rare.

• Serve the sliced goose breast with no additional sides or sauces to keep it true to the carnivore diet.

• Drink plenty of water and stay hydrated when following a carnivore diet.

# 19. Rabbit stew

## Ingredient:

• 1 whole rabbit, cut into 8 pieces
• 2 cups beef or chicken broth
• Salt and pepper to taste

## Instructions:

1. Pat the rabbit pieces dry with paper towels and season generously with salt and pepper.

2. Heat a large, heavy•bottomed pot or Dutch oven over medium•high heat. Add the rabbit pieces and brown them on all sides, about 3•4 minutes per side.

3. Once the rabbit is browned, pour in the broth and bring the mixture to a simmer.

4. Reduce the heat to low, cover the pot, and let the stew simmer for 60•90 minutes, or until the rabbit is very tender and the meat is falling off the bone.

5. Remove the lid and continue simmering for an additional 10•15 minutes to allow the stew to thicken slightly.

6. Serve the rabbit stew warm, with the meat and broth.

Tips:
• Choose a fresh, high•quality rabbit for the best flavor and tenderness.

• Adjust the cooking time as needed, depending on the size and age of the rabbit.

• Serve the rabbit stew with no additional sides or sauces to keep it true to the carnivore diet.

• Drink plenty of water and stay hydrated when following a carnivore diet.

# 20. Oxtail stew

## Ingredient:

• 2 lbs oxtails, cut into 2•inch pieces
• 4 cups beef broth
• Salt and pepper to taste

## Instructions:

1. Pat the oxtail pieces dry with paper towels and season generously with salt and pepper.

2. Heat a large, heavy•bottomed pot or Dutch oven over medium•high heat. Add the oxtail pieces and brown them on all sides, about 3•4 minutes per side.

3. Once the oxtail is browned, pour in the beef broth and bring the mixture to a simmer.

4. Reduce the heat to low, cover the pot, and let the stew simmer for 2•3 hours, or until the meat is very tender and falling off the bone.

5. Remove the lid and continue simmering for an additional 15•20 minutes to allow the stew to thicken slightly.

6. Serve the oxtail stew warm, with the meat and rich, flavorful broth.

Tips:
• Choose high•quality, fresh oxtails for the best flavor and tenderness.

• Adjust the cooking time as needed, depending on the size and quality of the oxtails.

• Serve the oxtail stew with no additional sides or sauces to keep it true to the carnivore diet.

• Drink plenty of water and stay hydrated when following a carnivore diet.

# 21. Pork belly slices

## Ingredient:

• 1 lb pork belly, cut into 1/2•inch thick slices
• Salt and pepper to taste

## Instructions:

1. Pat the pork belly slices dry with paper towels and season generously with salt and pepper on both sides.

2. Heat a cast•iron skillet or heavy•bottomed pan over medium•high heat. Once the pan is hot, add the pork belly slices in a single layer and sear for 3•4 minutes per side, or until the skin is crispy and golden brown.

3. Reduce the heat to medium•low and continue cooking the pork belly slices, flipping occasionally, until they are cooked through, about 10•12 minutes total.

4. Transfer the pork belly slices to a plate and let them rest for 5 minutes before serving.

Tips:
• Choose high•quality, fresh pork belly for the best flavor and texture.

• Avoid overcooking the pork belly, as it can become tough and dry if cooked past well•done.

• Serve the pork belly slices with no additional sides or sauces to keep it true to the carnivore diet.

• Drink plenty of water and stay hydrated when following a carnivore diet.

# 22. Lamb shank

## Ingredient:

• 2 lamb shanks
• Salt and pepper to taste

## Instructions:

1. Pat the lamb shanks dry with paper towels and season generously with salt and pepper on all sides.

2. Preheat your oven to 325°F (165°C).

3. Heat a large, oven•safe pot or Dutch oven over medium•high heat. Add the lamb shanks and sear them on all sides until a nice brown crust forms, about 3•4 minutes per side.

4. Once the shanks are seared, transfer the pot to the preheated oven and roast for 2•3 hours, or until the meat is very tender and falling off the bone.

5. Remove the pot from the oven and let the lamb shanks rest for 10•15 minutes before serving.

Tips:
• Choose high•quality, fresh lamb shanks for the best flavor and tenderness.

• Adjust the cooking time as needed, depending on the size and thickness of the shanks.

• Serve the lamb shanks with no additional sides or sauces to keep it true to the carnivore diet.

• Drink plenty of water and stay hydrated when following a carnivore diet.

# 23. Liver (beef, chicken, pork)

## Ingredient:

• 1 lb liver (beef, chicken, or pork), sliced into 1/4•inch thick pieces
• Salt and pepper to taste
• Butter or tallow for cooking

## Instructions:

1. Pat the liver slices dry with paper towels and season generously with salt and pepper on both sides.

2. Heat a large skillet over medium•high heat and add a small amount of butter or tallow.

3. Working in batches if needed, add the liver slices to the hot pan and sear for 2•3 minutes per side, or until a nice brown crust forms.

4. Reduce the heat to medium•low and continue cooking the liver, flipping occasionally, until it is cooked through but still slightly pink in the center, about 5•7 minutes total.

5. Transfer the seared liver to a plate and let it rest for 5 minutes before serving.

Tips:
• Choose high•quality, fresh liver for the best flavor and texture.

• Avoid overcooking the liver, as it can become tough and dry if cooked past medium.

• Serve the seared liver with no additional sides or sauces to keep it true to the carnivore diet.

• Drink plenty of water and stay hydrated when following a carnivore diet.

# 24. Kidneys (beef, lamb)

## Ingredient:

• 1 lb beef or lamb kidneys, trimmed and sliced into 1/4•inch thick pieces
• Salt and pepper to taste
• Butter or tallow for cooking

## Instructions:

1. Pat the kidney slices dry with paper towels and season generously with salt and pepper on both sides.

2. Heat a large skillet over medium•high heat and add a small amount of butter or tallow.

3. Working in batches if needed, add the kidney slices to the hot pan and sauté for 2•3 minutes per side, or until they are lightly browned.

4. Reduce the heat to medium•low and continue cooking the kidneys, stirring occasionally, until they are cooked through but still slightly pink in the center, about 5•7 minutes total.

5. Transfer the sautéed kidneys to a plate and let them rest for 5 minutes before serving.

Tips:
• Choose high•quality, fresh kidneys for the best flavor and texture.

• Avoid overcooking the kidneys, as they can become tough and rubbery if cooked past medium.

• Serve the sautéed kidneys with no additional sides or sauces to keep it true to the carnivore diet.

• Drink plenty of water and stay hydrated when following a carnivore diet.

# 25. Bone marrow

## Ingredient:

• 4 beef marrow bones, about 3•4 inches long
• Salt and pepper to taste

## Instructions:

1. Preheat your oven to 400°F (200°C).

2. Rinse the marrow bones and pat them dry with paper towels. Season the bones generously with salt and pepper.

3. Place the seasoned bones on a baking sheet or in a shallow roasting pan. Roast for 15•20 minutes, or until the marrow is soft and starting to ooze out of the bones.

4. Remove the bones from the oven and let them rest for 5 minutes.

5. Using a small spoon or fork, scoop the roasted marrow out of the bones and onto a plate or serving board.

6. Serve the roasted bone marrow immediately, while it's still hot and creamy.

Tips:
• Choose high•quality, fresh beef marrow bones for the best flavor and texture.

• Avoid overcooking the marrow, as it can become dry and tough if left in the oven too long.

• Serve the roasted bone marrow with no additional sides or sauces to keep it true to the carnivore diet.

• Drink plenty of water and stay hydrated when following a carnivore diet.

# 26. Pork ribs

## Ingredient:

• 2 lbs pork ribs, cut into individual ribs
• Salt and pepper to taste

## Instructions:

1. Pat the pork ribs dry with paper towels and season generously with salt and pepper on all sides.

2. Preheat your oven to 375°F (190°C).

3. Heat a large, oven•safe skillet or baking sheet over medium•high heat. Add the seasoned pork ribs in a single layer and sear for 2•3 minutes per side, or until they develop a nice brown crust.

4. Transfer the skillet or baking sheet to the preheated oven and roast the ribs for 45•60 minutes, or until the meat is tender and pulling away from the bone.

5. Remove the ribs from the oven and let them rest for 5•10 minutes before serving.

Tips:
• Choose high•quality, fresh pork ribs for the best flavor and tenderness.

• Adjust the cooking time as needed, depending on the thickness and size of the ribs.

• Serve the pork ribs with no additional sides or sauces to keep it true to the carnivore diet.

• Drink plenty of water and stay hydrated when following a carnivore diet.

# 27. Beef short ribs

## Ingredient:

• 2 lbs beef short ribs
• Salt and pepper to taste

## Instructions:

1. Pat the beef short ribs dry with paper towels and season generously with salt and pepper on all sides.

2. Preheat your oven to 325°F (165°C).

3. Heat a large, oven•safe pot or Dutch oven over medium•high heat. Add the seasoned short ribs and sear them on all sides until a nice brown crust forms, about 3•4 minutes per side.

4. Once the ribs are seared, transfer the pot to the preheated oven and roast for 2•3 hours, or until the meat is very tender and falling off the bone.

5. Remove the pot from the oven and let the short ribs rest for 10•15 minutes before serving.

Tips:
• Choose high•quality, fresh beef short ribs for the best flavor and tenderness.

• Adjust the cooking time as needed, depending on the size and thickness of the ribs.

• Serve the beef short ribs with no additional sides or sauces to keep it true to the carnivore diet.

• Drink plenty of water and stay hydrated when following a carnivore diet.

# 28. Beef tongue

## Ingredient:

• 1 beef tongue, trimmed and cleaned
• 1 onion, diced
• 3 carrots, peeled and diced
• 3 celery stalks, diced
• 6 cloves garlic, minced
• 2 bay leaves
• 2 sprigs fresh thyme
• 1 cup red wine
• 4 cups beef broth
• Salt and pepper to taste

## Instructions:

1. Place the beef tongue in a large pot and cover with water. Bring to a boil over high heat, then reduce to a simmer and cook for 2•3 hours, until the tongue is very tender.

2. Drain the tongue and let it cool slightly. Once cool enough to handle, peel off the tough outer skin. Slice or cube the tongue meat.

3. In a large Dutch oven or heavy•bottomed pot, heat a few tablespoons of olive oil over medium heat. Add the diced onion, carrots, and celery. Cook for 8•10 minutes, stirring occasionally, until the vegetables are softened.

4. Add the minced garlic and cook for 1 minute more, until fragrant.

5. Pour in the red wine and use a wooden spoon to scrape up any browned bits from the bottom of the pot. Let the wine come to a simmer and cook for 2•3 minutes.

6. Add the cooked and peeled beef tongue, bay leaves, thyme, and beef broth. Season with salt and pepper.

7. Bring the mixture to a boil, then reduce the heat to low, cover the pot, and let the tongue braise for 1.5•2 hours, until very tender.

8. Remove the bay leaves and thyme sprigs. Taste and adjust seasoning as needed.

9. Serve the braised beef tongue warm, over mashed potatoes, egg noodles, or with crusty bread. Garnish with chopped parsley if desired

# 29. Beef heart

## Ingredient:

- 1 beef heart, trimmed of any connective tissue and cut into 1•inch cubes
- 2 tablespoons olive oil
- 1 onion, diced
- 3 cloves garlic, minced
- 1 cup red wine
- 2 cups beef broth
- 2 bay leaves
- 2 sprigs fresh thyme
- 1 teaspoon dried oregano
- Salt and pepper to taste

## Instructions:

1. Pat the beef heart cubes dry with paper towels and season generously with salt and pepper.

2. In a large Dutch oven or heavy•bottomed pot, heat the olive oil over medium•high heat. Working in batches if needed, sear the beef heart cubes on all sides until browned, about 2•3 minutes per side. Transfer the seared meat to a plate.

3. Reduce the heat to medium and add the onions to the pot. Cook for 5•7 minutes, stirring occasionally, until softened and lightly browned.

4. Add the garlic and cook for 1 minute more, until fragrant.

5. Pour in the red wine and use a wooden spoon to scrape up any browned bits from the bottom of the pot. Let the wine come to a simmer and cook for 2•3 minutes.

6. Return the seared beef heart to the pot and add the beef broth, bay leaves, thyme, and oregano. Bring to a boil.

7. Once boiling, reduce the heat to low, cover the pot, and let the beef heart braise for 1.5•2 hours, until very tender.

8. Remove the bay leaves and thyme sprigs. Taste and adjust seasoning with salt and pepper as needed.

9. Serve the braised beef heart warm, over mashed potatoes, egg noodles, or with crusty bread.

# 30. Chicken liver pate

## Ingredient:

- 1 lb chicken livers, trimmed of any connective tissue
- 1/2 cup unsalted butter, softened
- 1/4 cup heavy cream
- 2 tablespoons brandy or cognac
- 1 teaspoon Dijon mustard
- 1 teaspoon fresh thyme leaves
- 1/2 teaspoon salt
- 1/4 teaspoon white pepper

## Instructions:

1. In a large skillet, cook the chicken livers over medium·high heat until browned on the outside but still slightly pink in the center, about 5·7 minutes. Transfer to a food processor.

2. Add the softened butter, heavy cream, brandy, Dijon mustard, thyme, salt, and white pepper to the food processor. Blend until smooth and creamy, scraping down the sides as needed.

3. Transfer the pâté to a serving dish or ramekins. Cover and refrigerate for at least 2 hours, or up to 5 days.

4. Serve the pâté chilled, with crackers, toasted bread, or crostini. Garnish with additional fresh thyme sprigs if desired.

Tips:
- For a smoother texture, pass the pâté through a fine mesh sieve after blending.

- Try adding a splash of port or madeira wine for extra flavor.

- Refrigerate any leftover pâté in an airtight container for up to 1 week.

# 31. Chicken gizzards

## Ingredient:

- 1 lb chicken gizzards, cleaned and trimmed
- 2 tablespoons olive oil
- 1 onion, diced
- 3 cloves garlic, minced
- 1 teaspoon paprika
- 1/2 teaspoon dried thyme
- 1/4 teaspoon cayenne pepper (optional)
- Salt and pepper to taste
- 2 tablespoons chopped parsley (for garnish)

## Instructions:

1. Rinse the chicken gizzards under cold water and pat them dry thoroughly with paper towels. Trim off any tough connective tissue.

2. In a large skillet, heat the olive oil over medium•high heat. Add the gizzards in a single layer and sear for 2•3 minutes per side until browned on the outside.

3. Reduce the heat to medium and add the diced onion to the pan. Cook for 5•7 minutes, stirring occasionally, until the onions are softened.

4. Add the minced garlic, paprika, thyme, and cayenne (if using). Cook for 1 minute, stirring constantly, until fragrant.

5. Pour in 1/4 cup of water or chicken broth and use a wooden spoon to scrape up any browned bits from the bottom of the pan.

6. Reduce the heat to low, cover the pan, and let the gizzards simmer for 45 minutes to 1 hour, until very tender.

7. Uncover the pan and let any excess liquid evaporate, if needed. Season the gizzards with salt and pepper to taste.

8. Transfer the sautéed chicken gizzards to a serving dish and garnish with the chopped parsley.

Serve the gizzards warm, as a main dish or appetizer. They pair well with rice, mashed potatoes, or crusty bread.

# 32. Pork sausage

## Ingredient:

- 2 lbs ground pork
- 1 tsp sea salt
- 1 tsp black pepper
- 1 tsp ground sage
- 1/2 tsp ground fennel seed
- 1/4 tsp ground nutmeg
- 1/4 tsp ground cloves

## Instructions:

1. In a large bowl, combine the ground pork, salt, pepper, sage, fennel seed, nutmeg, and cloves. Mix well until the seasonings are evenly distributed.

2. Form the seasoned pork into patties or links, depending on your preference.

3. Heat a large skillet over medium•high heat. Add the sausage patties or links and cook for 4•5 minutes per side, until browned and cooked through.

4. Alternatively, you can bake the sausages in the oven at 400°F for 20•25 minutes, flipping halfway, until fully cooked.

5. Serve the carnivore pork sausages warm, as part of a carnivore•friendly breakfast or meal.

Tips:
- For a smoother texture, you can grind the pork yourself using a meat grinder or food processor.
- Adjust the seasoning amounts to your taste preferences.
- Store any leftover cooked sausages in an airtight container in the refrigerator for up to 4 days.

This pork sausage recipe is perfect for a carnivore diet, as it is high in protein and fat, and contains no carbohydrates or plant•based ingredients. It's a great option for women following a carnivore lifestyle.

# 33. Lamb kebabs

## Ingredient:

• 2 lbs lamb, cut into 1•inch cubes
• 1 tsp sea salt
• 1/2 tsp black pepper
• 1/2 tsp ground cumin
• 1/4 tsp ground cinnamon
• 1/4 tsp ground cardamom
• Lemon wedges, for serving (optional)

## Instructions:

1. In a large bowl, combine the cubed lamb, salt, pepper, cumin, cinnamon, and cardamom. Toss to coat the lamb evenly with the spices.

2. Thread the seasoned lamb cubes onto metal or wooden skewers, leaving a small space between each piece.

3. Preheat your grill or grill pan to medium•high heat.

4. Grill the lamb kebabs for 8•10 minutes, turning occasionally, until the lamb is cooked to your desired doneness. For medium•rare, the internal temperature should reach 130°F.

5. Transfer the grilled lamb kebabs to a serving platter. Serve immediately, with lemon wedges on the side if desired.

Tips:
• Soak wooden skewers in water for 30 minutes before using to prevent them from burning.

• You can also broil the lamb kebabs in the oven for 8•10 minutes, turning halfway through.

• For extra flavor, you can marinate the lamb in a mixture of olive oil, lemon juice, and the spices for 30 minutes to 1 hour before threading onto the skewers.

This carnivore•friendly lamb kebab recipe is high in protein and healthy fats, making it an excellent choice for women following a carnivore diet. The blend of spices adds depth of flavor without any carbohydrates or plant•based ingredients.

# 34. Beef kebabs

## Ingredient:

• 2 lbs beef sirloin or tenderloin, cut into 1•inch cubes
• 1 tsp sea salt
• 1/2 tsp black pepper
• 1/2 tsp garlic powder
• 1/4 tsp smoked paprika
• Lemon wedges, for serving (optional)

## Instructions:

1. In a large bowl, combine the cubed beef, salt, pepper, garlic powder, and smoked paprika. Toss to coat the beef evenly with the seasonings.

2. Thread the seasoned beef cubes onto metal or wooden skewers, leaving a small space between each piece.

3. Preheat your grill or grill pan to medium•high heat.

4. Grill the beef kebabs for 8•10 minutes, turning occasionally, until the beef is cooked to your desired doneness. For medium•rare, the internal temperature should reach 130°F.

5. Transfer the grilled beef kebabs to a serving platter. Serve immediately, with lemon wedges on the side if desired.

Tips:
• Soak wooden skewers in water for 30 minutes before using to prevent them from burning.

• You can also broil the beef kebabs in the oven for 8•10 minutes, turning halfway through.

• For extra flavor, you can marinate the beef in a mixture of olive oil, lemon juice, and the seasonings for 30 minutes to 1 hour before threading onto the skewers.

This carnivore•friendly beef kebab recipe is high in protein and healthy fats, making it an excellent choice for women following a carnivore diet. The simple seasoning blend allows the natural flavor of the beef to shine.

# 35. Beef jerky (sugar•free)

## Ingredient:

• 2 lbs beef (such as flank steak or top round), sliced into 1/4•inch thick strips
• 2 tsp sea salt
• 1 tsp black pepper
• 1 tsp garlic powder
• 1 tsp onion powder
• 1/2 tsp smoked paprika
• 1/4 tsp cayenne pepper (optional, for a spicy kick)

## Instructions:

1. In a large bowl, combine the sliced beef strips with the sea salt, black pepper, garlic powder, onion powder, smoked paprika, and cayenne (if using). Toss to coat the beef evenly with the seasonings.

2. Arrange the seasoned beef strips in a single layer on dehydrator trays or baking sheets lined with parchment paper. Make sure the strips are not touching each other.

3. If using a dehydrator, dehydrate the beef jerky at 155°F for 6•8 hours, or until the jerky is dry and leathery, but still pliable.

4. If using an oven, preheat it to the lowest temperature setting, usually around 135°F. Place the baking sheets in the oven and let the beef jerky dry for 6•8 hours, flipping the strips halfway through, until the jerky is dry and leathery.

5. Once the jerky is fully dried, let it cool completely before storing.

6. Store the sugar•free beef jerky in an airtight container or resealable plastic bag at room temperature for up to 2 weeks.

Tips:
• For a more uniform thickness, partially freeze the beef before slicing.
• Adjust the spices to your taste preferences.
• You can also use a smoker to add a delicious smoky flavor to the jerky.

This sugar•free beef jerky is perfect for a carnivore diet, as it is high in protein and healthy fats, with no added sugars or carbohydrates. Enjoy this satisfying and nutritious snack!

# 36. Pork tenderloin

## Ingredient:

• 1 lb pork tenderloin, trimmed of any silver skin
• 1 tsp sea salt
• 1/2 tsp black pepper
• 1/2 tsp garlic powder
• 1/4 tsp ground cumin
• 1/4 tsp paprika
• 2 tbsp unsalted butter or ghee

## Instructions:

1. Preheat your oven to 400°F.

2. In a small bowl, combine the sea salt, black pepper, garlic powder, cumin, and paprika. Rub the seasoning mixture all over the pork tenderloin, making sure to coat it evenly.

3. In a large, oven•safe skillet or cast•iron pan, melt the butter or ghee over medium•high heat.

4. Sear the pork tenderloin on all sides until a nice brown crust forms, about 2•3 minutes per side.

5. Transfer the skillet to the preheated oven and roast the pork tenderloin for 15•20 minutes, or until the internal temperature reaches 145°F for medium•rare, or 160°F for medium.

6. Remove the pork tenderloin from the oven and let it rest for 5•10 minutes before slicing. Slice the pork tenderloin into 1/2•inch thick medallions and serve immediately.

Tips:
• For a more tender pork tenderloin, you can brine it in a saltwater solution for 30 minutes to 1 hour before cooking.
• Adjust the cooking time based on the thickness of your pork tenderloin and your desired level of doneness.
• Serve the pork tenderloin with a side of roasted vegetables or a simple salad for a complete carnivore•friendly meal.

This carnivore•friendly pork tenderloin recipe is high in protein and healthy fats, making it an excellent choice for women following a carnivore diet. The simple seasoning blend allows the natural flavor of the pork to shine.

# 37. Beef brisket

## Ingredient:

• 3•4 lb beef brisket, trimmed of excess fat
• 2 tsp sea salt
• 1 tsp black pepper
• 1 tsp garlic powder
• 1 tsp onion powder
• 1/2 tsp smoked paprika
• 1/4 cup beef tallow or ghee, for cooking

## Instructions:

1. Preheat your oven to 300°F.

2. In a small bowl, combine the sea salt, black pepper, garlic powder, onion powder, and smoked paprika. Rub the seasoning mixture all over the beef brisket, making sure to coat it evenly on all sides.

3. In a large, oven•safe Dutch oven or heavy•bottomed pot, melt the beef tallow or ghee over medium•high heat.

4. Sear the seasoned beef brisket on all sides until a nice brown crust forms, about 2•3 minutes per side.

5. Once seared, cover the pot with a tight•fitting lid and transfer it to the preheated oven.

6. Roast the beef brisket for 3•4 hours, or until it's fork•tender and the internal temperature reaches 195°F.

7. Remove the pot from the oven and let the brisket rest for 15•20 minutes before slicing against the grain into thin, tender slices.

Tips:
• For extra flavor, you can add a few sprigs of fresh thyme or rosemary to the pot during the braising process.
• If the brisket seems dry, you can baste it with the cooking juices every 30 minutes or so during the braising.
• Serve the sliced beef brisket with a side of roasted vegetables or a simple salad for a complete carnivore•friendly meal.

This carnivore•friendly beef brisket recipe is high in protein and healthy fats, making it an excellent choice for women following a carnivore diet. The long, slow cooking process ensures the brisket is tender and flavorful.

# 38. Lamb shoulder

## Ingredient:

• 3•4 lb lamb shoulder roast, bone•in or boneless
• 2 tsp sea salt
• 1 tsp black pepper
• 1 tsp dried rosemary
• 1/2 tsp ground cumin
• 1/4 tsp ground cinnamon
• 2 tbsp beef tallow or ghee, for cooking

## Instructions:

1. Preheat your oven to 325°F.

2. In a small bowl, combine the sea salt, black pepper, dried rosemary, ground cumin, and ground cinnamon. Rub the seasoning mixture all over the lamb shoulder, making sure to coat it evenly on all sides.

3. In a large, oven•safe Dutch oven or heavy•bottomed pot, heat the beef tallow or ghee over medium•high heat.

4. Sear the seasoned lamb shoulder on all sides until a nice brown crust forms, about 2•3 minutes per side.

5. Once seared, cover the pot with a tight•fitting lid and transfer it to the preheated oven.

6. Roast the lamb shoulder for 2.5•3.5 hours, or until the meat is fork•tender and the internal temperature reaches 195°F.

7. Remove the pot from the oven and let the lamb shoulder rest for 15•20 minutes before slicing or shredding the meat.

Tips:
• For extra flavor, you can add a few sprigs of fresh rosemary or thyme to the pot during the braising process.

• If the lamb shoulder seems dry, you can baste it with the cooking juices every 30 minutes or so during the braising.

• Serve the sliced or shredded lamb shoulder with a side of roasted vegetables or a simple salad for a complete carnivore•friendly meal.

# 39. Pork loin roast

## Ingredient:

- 3•4 lb pork loin roast, boneless
- 2 tsp sea salt
- 1 tsp black pepper
- 1 tsp garlic powder
- 1/2 tsp onion powder
- 1/4 tsp ground sage
- 2 tbsp beef tallow or ghee, for cooking

## Instructions:

1. Preheat your oven to 375°F.

2. In a small bowl, combine the sea salt, black pepper, garlic powder, onion powder, and ground sage. Rub the seasoning mixture all over the pork loin roast, making sure to coat it evenly on all sides.

3. In a large, oven•safe Dutch oven or heavy•bottomed pot, heat the beef tallow or ghee over medium•high heat.

4. Sear the seasoned pork loin roast on all sides until a nice brown crust forms, about 2•3 minutes per side.

5. Once seared, cover the pot with a tight•fitting lid and transfer it to the preheated oven.

6. Roast the pork loin for 45•60 minutes, or until the internal temperature reaches 145°F for medium•rare, or 160°F for medium.

7. Remove the pot from the oven and let the pork loin rest for 10•15 minutes before slicing. Slice the pork loin roast into 1/2•inch thick medallions and serve immediately.

Tips:
- For extra flavor, you can add a few sprigs of fresh rosemary or thyme to the pot during the roasting process.

- If the pork loin seems dry, you can baste it with the cooking juices every 20 minutes or so during the roasting.

- Serve the sliced pork loin roast with a side of roasted vegetables or a simple salad for a complete carnivore•friendly meal.

# 40. Chicken breast

## Ingredient:

• 4 (6 oz) boneless, skinless chicken breasts
• 1 tsp sea salt
• 1/2 tsp black pepper
• 1/2 tsp garlic powder
• 2 tbsp unsalted butter or ghee

## Instructions:

1. Preheat your oven to 400°F.

2. Pat the chicken breasts dry with paper towels and season them evenly with the sea salt, black pepper, and garlic powder.

3. In a large, oven•safe skillet or cast•iron pan, melt the butter or ghee over medium•high heat.

4. Once the butter is hot, carefully place the chicken breasts in the pan. Sear for 3•4 minutes per side, or until a nice golden•brown crust forms.

5. Transfer the skillet to the preheated oven and roast the chicken for 12•15 minutes, or until the internal temperature reaches 165°F.

6. Remove the skillet from the oven and let the chicken rest for 5 minutes before serving.

Tips:
• For extra flavor, you can rub the chicken breasts with a blend of dried herbs, such as rosemary, thyme, or oregano, before searing.

• If you don't have an oven•safe skillet, you can transfer the seared chicken breasts to a parchment•lined baking sheet before roasting in the oven.

• Serve the chicken breasts with a side of roasted vegetables or a simple salad for a complete carnivore•friendly meal.

This carnivore•friendly chicken breast recipe is high in protein and low in carbohydrates, making it an excellent choice for women following a carnivore diet. The simple seasoning and cooking method ensure the chicken remains juicy and flavorful.

# 41. Salmon fillet

## Ingredient:

• 4 (6 oz) salmon fillets, skin•on
• 1 tsp sea salt
• 1/2 tsp black pepper
• 1/2 tsp garlic powder
• 2 tbsp unsalted butter or ghee

## Instructions:

1. Preheat your oven to 400°F.

2. Pat the salmon fillets dry with paper towels and season them evenly with the sea salt, black pepper, and garlic powder.

3. In a large, oven•safe skillet or cast•iron pan, melt the butter or ghee over medium•high heat.

4. Once the butter is hot, carefully place the salmon fillets skin•side down in the pan. Sear for 3•4 minutes, or until the skin is crispy and golden brown.

5. Flip the salmon fillets and transfer the skillet to the preheated oven.

6. Roast the salmon for 8•12 minutes, or until it flakes easily with a fork and the internal temperature reaches 145°F.

7. Remove the skillet from the oven and let the salmon rest for 5 minutes before serving.

Tips:
• For extra flavor, you can add a squeeze of lemon juice or a sprinkle of chopped fresh dill over the salmon before serving.

• If you don't have an oven•safe skillet, you can transfer the seared salmon fillets to a parchment•lined baking sheet before roasting in the oven.

• Serve the salmon fillets with a side of roasted vegetables or a simple salad for a complete carnivore•friendly meal.

This carnivore•friendly salmon recipe is high in protein, healthy fats, and essential nutrients, making it an excellent choice for women following a carnivore diet. The simple seasoning allows the natural flavor of the salmon to shine.

# 42. Tuna steak

## Ingredient:

• 4 (6 oz) tuna steaks, about 1•inch thick
• 1 tsp sea salt
• 1/2 tsp black pepper
• 1/2 tsp garlic powder
• 2 tbsp avocado oil or ghee

## Instructions:

1. Pat the tuna steaks dry with paper towels and season them evenly with the sea salt, black pepper, and garlic powder.

2. In a large, heavy•bottomed skillet or cast•iron pan, heat the avocado oil or ghee over high heat.

3. When the oil is shimmering, carefully add the seasoned tuna steaks to the pan. Sear for 2•3 minutes per side, or until a nice crust forms on the outside but the center is still rare to medium•rare.

4. Remove the tuna steaks from the pan and let them rest for 5 minutes before serving.

Tips:
• For a more well•done tuna steak, you can sear the steaks for an additional 1•2 minutes per side.

• Avoid overcooking the tuna, as it can become dry and tough.

• Serve the tuna steaks immediately, with a side of roasted vegetables or a simple salad for a complete carnivore•friendly meal.

• You can also top the tuna steaks with a pat of butter or a drizzle of lemon juice for extra flavor.

This carnivore•friendly tuna steak recipe is high in protein, healthy fats, and essential nutrients, making it an excellent choice for women following a carnivore diet. The simple seasoning allows the natural flavor of the tuna to shine

# 43. Sardines

**Ingredient:**

- 1 (4.25 oz) can of sardines in olive oil or water, drained
- 1/2 tsp sea salt
- 1/4 tsp black pepper
- Lemon wedges, for serving (optional)

**Instructions:**

1. Drain the sardines from the can and transfer them to a small bowl.

2. Season the sardines with the sea salt and black pepper, gently tossing to coat them evenly.

3. Serve the seasoned sardines immediately, either on their own or with lemon wedges on the side.

Tips:
- For extra flavor, you can add a sprinkle of dried herbs, such as oregano or parsley, to the sardines.

- If you prefer, you can mash the sardines with a fork and serve them on a bed of greens or with a side of roasted vegetables.

- Canned sardines are a convenient and nutrient•dense option for a carnivore diet, as they are high in protein, healthy fats, and essential vitamins and minerals.

This simple sardine recipe is perfect for a carnivore diet, as it is high in protein and healthy fats, with no carbohydrates or plant•based ingredients. Sardines are an excellent source of omega•3 fatty acids, which are important for overall health and well•being.

# 44. Mackerel

## Ingredient:

• 4 (6 oz) mackerel fillets, skin•on
• 1 tsp sea salt
• 1/2 tsp black pepper
• 1 tbsp avocado oil or ghee

## Instructions:

1. Pat the mackerel fillets dry with paper towels and season them evenly with the sea salt and black pepper.

2. In a large, non•stick skillet, heat the avocado oil or ghee over medium•high heat.

3. When the oil is hot, carefully place the mackerel fillets skin•side down in the pan. Sear for 3•4 minutes, or until the skin is crispy and golden brown.

4. Flip the mackerel fillets and continue cooking for an additional 2•3 minutes, or until the fish flakes easily with a fork and is cooked through.

5. Remove the mackerel fillets from the pan and serve immediately.

Tips:
• For extra flavor, you can squeeze a bit of lemon juice over the mackerel before serving.

• Mackerel is a highly nutritious fish, rich in omega•3 fatty acids, protein, and essential vitamins and minerals.

• Serve the mackerel fillets with a side of roasted vegetables or a simple salad for a complete carnivore•friendly meal.

This simple mackerel recipe is perfect for a carnivore diet, as it is high in protein and healthy fats, with no carbohydrates or plant•based ingredients. The crispy skin and tender, flavorful flesh make this an excellent choice for a satisfying and nutritious meal.

# 45. Halibut

## Ingredient:

• 4 (6 oz) halibut fillets, skin•on
• 1 tsp sea salt
• 1/2 tsp black pepper
• 1/2 tsp garlic powder
• 2 tbsp unsalted butter or ghee

## Instructions:

1. Pat the halibut fillets dry with paper towels and season them evenly with the sea salt, black pepper, and garlic powder.

2. In a large, non•stick skillet, melt the butter or ghee over medium•high heat.

3. When the butter is hot and foaming, carefully place the seasoned halibut fillets skin•side down in the pan. Sear for 3•4 minutes, or until the skin is crispy and golden brown.

4. Flip the halibut fillets and continue cooking for an additional 4•6 minutes, or until the fish flakes easily with a fork and is cooked through.

5. Remove the halibut fillets from the pan and serve immediately.

Tips:
• For extra flavor, you can squeeze a bit of lemon juice over the halibut before serving.

• Halibut is a lean, flaky white fish that is an excellent source of protein and essential nutrients, making it a great choice for a carnivore diet.

• Serve the halibut fillets with a side of roasted vegetables or a simple salad for a complete carnivore•friendly meal.

This carnivore•friendly halibut recipe is high in protein, low in carbohydrates, and rich in healthy fats, making it an excellent choice for women following a carnivore diet. The simple seasoning and cooking method allow the natural flavor of the halibut to shine.

# 46. Cod fillet

## Ingredient:

- 4 (6 oz) cod fillets, skin•on
- 1 tsp sea salt
- 1/2 tsp black pepper
- 1/2 tsp paprika
- 2 tbsp unsalted butter or ghee

## Instructions:

1. Preheat your oven to 400°F.

2. Pat the cod fillets dry with paper towels and season them evenly with the sea salt, black pepper, and paprika.

3. In a large, oven•safe skillet or cast•iron pan, melt the butter or ghee over medium•high heat.

4. When the butter is hot, carefully place the seasoned cod fillets skin•side down in the pan. Sear for 2•3 minutes, or until the skin is crispy and golden brown.

5. Flip the cod fillets and transfer the skillet to the preheated oven.

6. Roast the cod for 8•12 minutes, or until the fish flakes easily with a fork and the internal temperature reaches 145°F.

7. Remove the skillet from the oven and let the cod rest for 5 minutes before serving.

Tips:
- For extra flavor, you can add a squeeze of lemon juice or a sprinkle of chopped fresh parsley over the cod before serving.

- If you don't have an oven•safe skillet, you can transfer the seared cod fillets to a parchment•lined baking sheet before roasting in the oven.

- Serve the cod fillets with a side of roasted vegetables or a simple salad for a complete carnivore•friendly meal.

This carnivore•friendly cod recipe is high in protein, low in carbohydrates, and rich in essential nutrients, making it an excellent choice for women following a carnivore diet. The simple seasoning and cooking method ensure the cod remains moist and flavorful

# 47. Swordfish steak

**Ingredient:**

• 4 (6 oz) swordfish steaks, about 1•inch thick
• 1 tsp sea salt
• 1/2 tsp black pepper
• 1/2 tsp garlic powder
• 2 tbsp avocado oil or ghee

**Instructions:**

1. Pat the swordfish steaks dry with paper towels and season them evenly with the sea salt, black pepper, and garlic powder.

2. In a large, heavy•bottomed skillet or cast•iron pan, heat the avocado oil or ghee over high heat.

3. When the oil is shimmering, carefully add the seasoned swordfish steaks to the pan. Sear for 3•4 minutes per side, or until a nice crust forms on the outside but the center is still slightly translucent.

4. Reduce the heat to medium•low and continue cooking the swordfish for an additional 2•3 minutes per side, or until the fish is cooked through and flakes easily with a fork.

5. Remove the swordfish steaks from the pan and let them rest for 5 minutes before serving.

Tips:
• Avoid overcooking the swordfish, as it can become dry and tough. The center should still be slightly pink when the fish is done.

• For extra flavor, you can baste the swordfish with a bit of melted butter or ghee during the cooking process.

• Serve the swordfish steaks immediately, with a side of roasted vegetables or a simple salad for a complete carnivore•friendly meal.

This carnivore•friendly swordfish recipe is high in protein, healthy fats, and essential nutrients, making it an excellent choice for women following a carnivore diet. The simple seasoning allows the natural flavor of the swordfish to shine.

# 48. Shrimp

## Ingredient:

- 1 lb raw, peeled and deveined shrimp
- 1 tsp sea salt
- 1/2 tsp black pepper
- 1/2 tsp garlic powder
- 2 tbsp unsalted butter or ghee

## Instructions:

1. Pat the shrimp dry with paper towels and season them evenly with the sea salt, black pepper, and garlic powder.

2. In a large skillet, melt the butter or ghee over medium•high heat.

3. When the butter is hot and foaming, carefully add the seasoned shrimp to the pan in a single layer.

4. Cook the shrimp for 2•3 minutes per side, or until they are opaque and cooked through.

5. Remove the shrimp from the pan and serve immediately.

Tips:
- For extra flavor, you can add a squeeze of lemon juice or a sprinkle of chopped fresh parsley over the shrimp before serving.

- Shrimp is a low•calorie, high•protein seafood that is an excellent choice for a carnivore diet.

- Serve the shrimp as a main dish, or use them as a protein•rich topping for a simple salad or roasted vegetables.

This carnivore•friendly shrimp recipe is quick and easy to prepare, making it a great option for a busy weeknight meal. The simple seasoning allows the natural sweetness of the shrimp to shine, while the butter or ghee adds a rich, satisfying flavor.

# 49. Lobster tail

## Ingredient:

• 4 (4•6 oz) lobster tails, thawed if frozen
• 2 tbsp unsalted butter, melted
• 1 tsp sea salt
• 1/2 tsp black pepper
• 1/2 tsp paprika
• Lemon wedges, for serving (optional)

## Instructions:

1. Preheat your oven to 400°F.

2. Using kitchen shears, carefully cut along the center of the lobster tails, leaving the bottom shell intact. Gently pull the lobster meat up and out of the shell, leaving the base attached.

3. In a small bowl, combine the melted butter, sea salt, black pepper, and paprika. Brush the seasoned butter mixture over the exposed lobster meat.

4. Arrange the prepared lobster tails on a parchment•lined baking sheet.

5. Roast the lobster tails in the preheated oven for 10•12 minutes, or until the meat is opaque and cooked through.

6. Remove the lobster tails from the oven and serve immediately, with lemon wedges on the side if desired.

Tips:
• For extra flavor, you can add a sprinkle of chopped fresh parsley or a squeeze of lemon juice over the cooked lobster tails.
• Lobster is a luxurious and nutrient•dense seafood that is an excellent choice for a carnivore diet, as it is high in protein and low in carbohydrates.
• Serve the lobster tails as a main dish, or use them as a protein•rich topping for a simple salad or roasted vegetables.

This carnivore•friendly lobster tail recipe is easy to prepare and showcases the natural sweetness and tenderness of the lobster meat. The simple seasoning allows the lobster to shine, making it a perfect choice for a special occasion or a indulgent weeknight meal.

# 50. Crab legs

## Ingredient:

• 2 lbs cooked and frozen king crab legs, thawed
• 4 tbsp unsalted butter, melted
• 1 tsp sea salt
• 1/2 tsp black pepper
• 1/2 tsp garlic powder
• Lemon wedges, for serving

## Instructions:

1. Preheat your oven to 400°F.

2. In a small bowl, combine the melted butter, sea salt, black pepper, and garlic powder. Stir to mix well.

3. Arrange the thawed crab legs on a large baking sheet or in a shallow baking dish. Brush the seasoned butter mixture over the crab legs, making sure to coat them evenly.

4. Roast the crab legs in the preheated oven for 10•12 minutes, or until heated through.

5. Remove the crab legs from the oven and serve immediately, with lemon wedges on the side.

Tips:
• For easier eating, you can crack the crab legs before roasting to make them easier to access the meat.

• Crab is a lean, protein•rich seafood that is an excellent choice for a carnivore diet. It's also a good source of essential vitamins and minerals.

• Serve the roasted crab legs as a main dish, or use them as a protein•rich topping for a simple salad or roasted vegetables.

This carnivore•friendly crab leg recipe is easy to prepare and showcases the sweet, delicate flavor of the crab meat. The simple seasoning allows the natural taste of the crab to shine, making it a perfect choice for a special occasion or a indulgent weeknight meal.

# 51. Scallops

## Ingredient:

- 1 lb sea scallops, patted dry
- 1 tsp sea salt
- 1/2 tsp black pepper
- 2 tbsp avocado oil or ghee

## Instructions:

1. Pat the scallops dry with paper towels and season them evenly with the sea salt and black pepper.

2. In a large, heavy•bottomed skillet or cast•iron pan, heat the avocado oil or ghee over high heat.

3. When the oil is shimmering, carefully add the seasoned scallops to the pan, making sure not to overcrowd them.

4. Sear the scallops for 2•3 minutes per side, or until a nice golden•brown crust forms and the centers are opaque. Remove the seared scallops from the pan and serve immediately.

Tips:
- Avoid overcooking the scallops, as they can become tough and rubbery. The centers should still be slightly translucent when they're done.

- For extra flavor, you can baste the scallops with a bit of melted butter or ghee during the cooking process.

- Serve the scallops as a main dish, or use them as a protein•rich topping for a simple salad or roasted vegetables.

This carnivore•friendly scallop recipe is high in protein, low in carbohydrates, and rich in healthy fats, making it an excellent choice for women following a carnivore diet. The simple seasoning and quick cooking method allow the natural sweetness and delicate texture of the scallops to shine.

# 52. Clams

## Ingredient:

• 2 lbs fresh clams, scrubbed clean
• 2 tbsp unsalted butter or ghee
• 1 tsp sea salt
• 1/2 tsp black pepper
• 1/4 cup dry white wine (optional)
• Lemon wedges, for serving

## Instructions:

1. In a large pot or Dutch oven, melt the butter or ghee over medium•high heat.

2. Add the cleaned clams to the pot and season them with the sea salt and black pepper.

3. If using, pour in the white wine and cover the pot with a tight•fitting lid.

4. Cook the clams for 5•7 minutes, shaking the pot occasionally, until the clams have opened up.

5. Discard any clams that did not open.

6. Carefully transfer the cooked clams to a serving bowl, making sure to include any juices that have accumulated in the pot. Serve the clams immediately, with lemon wedges on the side.

Tips:
• For extra flavor, you can add a few minced garlic cloves or a sprinkle of chopped parsley to the pot while the clams are cooking.

• Clams are a low•calorie, high•protein seafood that is an excellent choice for a carnivore diet. They are also a good source of essential minerals like iron and zinc.

• Serve the clams as a main dish, or use them as a protein•rich topping for a simple salad or roasted vegetables.

This carnivore•friendly clam recipe is quick and easy to prepare, making it a great option for a weeknight meal. The simple cooking method allows the natural briny flavor of the clams to shine, while the butter or ghee adds a rich, satisfying element.

# 53. Oysters

## Ingredient:

- 12 fresh oysters, shucked and on the half shell
- 2 tbsp unsalted butter, melted
- 1 tsp sea salt
- 1/2 tsp black pepper
- Lemon wedges, for serving

## Instructions:

1. Preheat your oven's broiler to high heat.

2. Arrange the shucked oysters on a baking sheet or in a shallow baking dish.

3. In a small bowl, combine the melted butter, sea salt, and black pepper. Stir to mix well.

4. Drizzle the seasoned butter over the oysters, making sure to coat them evenly.

5. Place the baking sheet or dish under the preheated broiler and cook for 2•3 minutes, or until the edges of the oysters start to curl and the butter is bubbly.

6. Remove the oysters from the oven and serve immediately, with lemon wedges on the side.

Tips:
• Be careful when shucking the oysters, as the shells can be sharp. Use an oyster shucker or a sturdy knife.

• For extra flavor, you can add a sprinkle of chopped fresh parsley or a squeeze of lemon juice over the oysters before serving.

• Oysters are a low•calorie, high•protein seafood that is an excellent choice for a carnivore diet. They are also a good source of essential minerals like zinc and selenium.

• Serve the broiled oysters as an appetizer or a light main dish.

This carnivore•friendly oyster recipe is quick and easy to prepare, and showcases the natural briny flavor of the oysters. The simple seasoning and broiling method allow the oysters to shine, making them a perfect choice for a special occasion or a indulgent weeknight meal.

# 54. Anchovies

## Ingredient:

- 8 oz spaghetti or linguine pasta
- 3 tbsp olive oil
- 3•4 anchovy fillets, finely chopped
- 3 cloves garlic, minced
- 1/4 tsp red pepper flakes (optional)
- 1/4 cup grated parmesan cheese
- 2 tbsp chopped parsley
- Salt and pepper to taste

## Instructions:

1. Bring a large pot of salted water to a boil. Cook the pasta according to package directions until al dente. Drain and reserve 1/2 cup of the pasta cooking water.

2. In a large skillet, heat the olive oil over medium heat. Add the chopped anchovies and garlic. Cook for 1•2 minutes, stirring frequently, until the anchovies have dissolved and the garlic is fragrant.

3. Add the cooked pasta to the skillet with the anchovy•garlic oil. Toss to coat the pasta. If the pasta seems dry, add a splash or two of the reserved pasta cooking water.

4. Remove from heat and stir in the red pepper flakes (if using), parmesan, and parsley. Season with salt and pepper to taste.

5. Serve the anchovy pasta immediately, garnished with extra parsley if desired.

The anchovies melt into the oil, creating a savory, umami•rich sauce that coats the pasta. Adjust the amount of anchovies to your taste preference. Enjoy!

# 55. Squid

## Ingredient:

- 1 lb fresh or frozen squid, cleaned and cut into rings or tentacles
- 2 tbsp avocado oil or ghee
- 1 tsp sea salt
- 1/2 tsp black pepper
- 1/2 tsp paprika
- Lemon wedges, for serving

## Instructions:

1. If using frozen squid, thaw it completely and pat it dry with paper towels.

2. In a large skillet or wok, heat the avocado oil or ghee over high heat.

3. Add the squid rings or tentacles to the hot oil and season them with the sea salt, black pepper, and paprika. Toss to coat the squid evenly.

4. Sauté the squid for 2•3 minutes, stirring frequently, until it is opaque and cooked through. Be careful not to overcook, as squid can become tough and rubbery.

5. Remove the skillet from the heat and transfer the sautéed squid to a serving plate.

6. Serve the squid immediately, with lemon wedges on the side.

Tips:
- For extra flavor, you can add a splash of dry white wine or a squeeze of lemon juice to the skillet during the cooking process.

- Squid is a lean, protein•rich seafood that is an excellent choice for a carnivore diet. It's also a good source of essential vitamins and minerals.

- Serve the sautéed squid as a main dish, or use it as a protein•rich topping for a simple salad or roasted vegetables.

This carnivore•friendly squid recipe is quick and easy to prepare, making it a great option for a weeknight meal. The simple seasoning and high•heat cooking method ensure the squid remains tender and flavorful, while the avocado oil or ghee adds a rich, satisfying element

# 56. Octopus

## Ingredient:

- 1 lb fresh octopus, cleaned and cut into 1/2·inch pieces
- 1 cup fresh lime juice (about 8·10 limes)
- 1/2 cup fresh orange juice
- 1 small red onion, thinly sliced
- 1 jalapeño, seeded and finely chopped
- 1 tomato, diced
- 1/4 cup chopped cilantro
- 1 avocado, diced
- Salt and pepper to taste

## Instructions:

1. In a large non·reactive bowl, combine the chopped octopus, lime juice, and orange juice. Cover and refrigerate for 2·3 hours, stirring occasionally, until the octopus is opaque and "cooked" through the acid in the citrus juices.

2. Drain any excess citrus juice from the octopus. Add the sliced red onion, jalapeño, tomato, cilantro, and avocado. Gently toss to combine.

3. Season the ceviche with salt and pepper to taste.

4. Serve the octopus ceviche chilled, with tortilla chips or tostones on the side.

The key to great ceviche is using the freshest, highest quality seafood you can find. The citrus juice "cooks" the octopus, giving it a firm, tender texture. Adjust the amount of jalapeño to your desired spice level. Enjoy this bright, refreshing octopus ceviche!

# 57. Beef liver and onions

## Ingredient:

- 1 lb beef liver, sliced into 1/4•inch thick pieces
- 2 tbsp tallow or avocado oil
- 1 large onion, thinly sliced
- 2 cloves garlic, minced
- 1 tsp dried thyme
- Salt and pepper to taste

## Instructions:

1. Pat the liver slices dry with paper towels and season generously with salt and pepper.

2. In a large skillet, heat the tallow or oil over medium•high heat. Working in batches if needed, sear the liver slices for 2•3 minutes per side until browned on the outside but still slightly pink in the center. Transfer the seared liver to a plate.

3. Reduce the heat to medium and add the sliced onions to the skillet. Cook for 5•7 minutes, stirring occasionally, until the onions are softened and starting to caramelize.

4. Add the minced garlic and thyme to the onions. Cook for 1 minute more, until fragrant.

5. Return the seared liver slices to the skillet with the onions. Cook for 2•3 minutes more, just to heat through.

6. Serve the beef liver and onions immediately. Optionally, you can top with a pat of grass•fed butter.

This recipe is perfect for a carnivore diet, as it provides high•quality protein, iron, and other essential nutrients from the beef liver. The onions add flavor and beneficial sulfur compounds. It's an excellent meal for women looking to support their health through a nutrient•dense, animal•based diet.

Enjoy!

# 58. Pate (various meats)

## Ingredient:

- 1 lb chicken livers, trimmed
- 1/2 cup unsalted butter, softened
- 1/4 cup brandy or cognac
- 2 tbsp heavy cream
- 1 tsp Dijon mustard
- 1/2 tsp salt
- 1/4 tsp white pepper

## Instructions:

1. In a skillet, cook the chicken livers over medium•high heat until browned on the outside but still pink in the center, about 5•7 minutes.

2. Transfer to a food processor and pulse until finely chopped.

3. Add the butter, brandy, cream, mustard, salt and pepper. Process until smooth and creamy. Transfer to ramekins or a terrine and refrigerate for at least 2 hours before serving.

### Duck Liver Pâté
### *Ingredients:*
- 1 lb duck livers, trimmed
- 1/2 cup unsalted butter, softened
- 1/4 cup Madeira wine
- 1 tsp cognac or brandy
- 1/2 tsp salt
- 1/4 tsp white pepper

### *Instructions:*
1. In a skillet, cook the duck livers over medium•high heat until browned on the outside but still pink in the center, about 5•7 minutes.

2. Transfer to a food processor and pulse until finely chopped.

3. Add the butter, Madeira, cognac, salt and pepper. Process until smooth and creamy.

4. Transfer to ramekins or a terrine and refrigerate for at least 2 hours before serving.

# 59. Heart skewers

## Ingredient:

- 1 lb beef heart, trimmed and cut into 1·inch cubes
- 2 tbsp tallow or avocado oil
- 1 tsp smoked paprika
- 1/2 tsp garlic powder
- 1/2 tsp onion powder
- Salt and pepper to taste
- Wooden or metal skewers

## Instructions:

1. In a medium bowl, toss the cubed beef heart with the tallow/oil, smoked paprika, garlic powder, onion powder, salt, and pepper until the heart pieces are evenly coated.

2. Thread the seasoned heart cubes onto skewers, leaving a little space between each piece.

3. Preheat your grill or grill pan to medium·high heat.

4. Grill the heart skewers for 2·3 minutes per side, until the outside is lightly charred and the inside is still slightly pink.

5. Serve the grilled heart skewers immediately, while hot.

Heart is an incredibly nutrient·dense organ meat that is an excellent addition to a carnivore diet, especially for women. It is rich in iron, vitamin B12, zinc, and other essential vitamins and minerals. The simple seasoning allows the natural flavor of the heart to shine.

Pair these heart skewers with a side salad or roasted vegetables for a complete, nourishing meal. Enjoy!

# 60. Kidney stew

## Ingredient:

- 1 lb lamb or beef kidneys, trimmed and cut into 1•inch pieces
- 2 tbsp all•purpose flour
- 2 tbsp vegetable oil
- 1 onion, diced
- 2 carrots, peeled and diced
- 2 celery stalks, diced
- 3 cloves garlic, minced
- 2 cups beef or chicken stock
- 1 cup red wine
- 2 bay leaves
- 2 sprigs fresh thyme
- 1 tsp Worcestershire sauce
- Salt and pepper to taste
- Chopped parsley for garnish

## Instructions:

1. Pat the kidney pieces dry and toss them with the flour until evenly coated.

2. Heat the oil in a large pot or Dutch oven over medium•high heat. Add the kidneys and cook, stirring occasionally, until browned on all sides, about 5 minutes. Transfer to a plate.

3. Add the onion, carrots, celery and garlic to the pot. Cook, stirring occasionally, until the vegetables are softened, about 5 minutes.

4. Pour in the stock and wine. Add the bay leaves, thyme, Worcestershire sauce, and season with salt and pepper.

5. Return the kidneys to the pot and bring to a boil. Reduce heat to low, cover and simmer for 45•60 minutes, until the kidneys are very tender.

6. Taste and adjust seasoning as needed. Garnish with chopped parsley before serving.

Serve the kidney stew over mashed potatoes, egg noodles or crusty bread to soak up the flavorful broth. Enjoy!

# 61. German bratwurst

**Ingredient:**

- 1 lb ground pork
- 1/2 lb ground veal
- 2 tsp salt
- 1 tsp white pepper
- 1 tsp ground nutmeg
- 1 tsp marjoram
- 1/2 tsp caraway seeds
- 1/4 cup milk
- Hog casings

**Instructions:**

1. Mix all ingredients except casings.

2. Chill mixture for 1 hour.

3. Stuff into hog casings.

4. Grill or pan•fry until internal temperature reaches 160°F (71°C).

# 62. Scrambled eggs

## Ingredient:

- 3 large eggs
- 1 tbsp unsalted butter or ghee
- 1/4 tsp salt
- 1/8 tsp black pepper

## Instructions:

1. Crack the eggs into a small bowl and beat them lightly with a fork until blended.

2. Melt the butter or ghee in a non•stick skillet over medium heat.

3. Pour the eggs into the skillet and let them sit for 10•15 seconds to set the bottom slightly.

4. Using a spatula, gently push the eggs from the edge of the pan towards the center, tilting the pan to allow the uncooked egg to flow to the edges.

5. Continue this gentle folding and pushing motion until the eggs are softly scrambled and cooked through, about 2•3 minutes total.

6. Remove from heat and season with salt and pepper.
7. Serve immediately.

Tips:
- Use high•quality, pasture•raised eggs for the best flavor and nutrition.

- Avoid overcooking the eggs to keep them tender and moist.

- You can add a sprinkle of grated cheese or a dollop of sour cream on top if desired.

- Pair with avocado, bacon, or sausage for a complete carnivore•friendly meal.

Enjoy your delicious and nutritious carnivore scrambled eggs!

# 63. Fried eggs

## Ingredient:

- 2 large eggs
- 1•2 tbsp butter or avocado oil
- Salt and pepper to taste

## Instructions:

1. Heat a small non•stick skillet over medium heat. Add the butter or oil and swirl to coat the bottom of the pan.

2. Crack the eggs directly into the hot pan, being careful not to break the yolks. Season with a pinch of salt and pepper.

3. Cook the eggs for 2•3 minutes, or until the whites are completely set but the yolks are still runny.

4. For over•easy eggs, flip the eggs carefully and cook for an additional 30 seconds to 1 minute.

5. For over•medium or over•hard, cook the flipped eggs for 1•2 minutes more, until the yolks reach your desired doneness.

6. Carefully transfer the fried eggs to a plate and serve immediately.

Tips:
• Use a non•stick pan and keep the heat at medium to prevent the eggs from sticking or overcooking.

• Basting the eggs with the hot fat can help the whites set without overcooking the yolks.

• For a crisper edge, let the eggs cook undisturbed until the whites are mostly set before flipping.

Fried eggs are a simple, versatile staple that can be enjoyed for breakfast, lunch, or dinner. Serve them on their own, on top of toast, or alongside other protein•rich foods for a satisfying meal. Enjoy!

# 64. Boiled eggs

## Ingredient:

• Large eggs

## Instructions:

1. Place the eggs in a single layer in a saucepan and cover with cold water by 1 inch.

2. Bring the water to a boil over high heat. Once the water reaches a full boil, remove the pan from the heat and cover.

3. Let the eggs sit in the hot water for the desired doneness:
• For soft•boiled eggs: 6•7 minutes
• For hard•boiled eggs: 12 minutes

4. Drain the hot water and cover the eggs with cold water to stop the cooking. Let sit for 2•3 minutes.

5. Peel the eggs and enjoy!

Tips:
• Use fresh, room temperature eggs for easier peeling.

• Add a teaspoon of baking soda to the water to help make the shells easier to peel.

• Serve the boiled eggs plain, or top with a sprinkle of salt and pepper.

• Hard•boiled eggs can be stored in the refrigerator for up to 1 week.

This simple boiled egg recipe is a great protein•packed option for a carnivore diet. Adjust the cooking time to your desired level of doneness. Enjoy!

# 65. Omelettes with various meat fillings

## Ingredient:

- 3 large eggs
- 1 tbsp unsalted butter or ghee
- Salt and pepper to taste
- Fillings (choose 1 or more):
  - Cooked bacon, crumbled
  - Cooked sausage, crumbled
  - Cooked ground beef or lamb
  - Shredded cooked chicken or turkey
  - Diced cooked ham
  - Grated cheese (optional)

## Instructions:

1. Crack the eggs into a small bowl and beat lightly with a fork until blended.

2. Melt the butter or ghee in a non•stick skillet over medium heat.

3. Pour the eggs into the skillet and let them sit for 10•15 seconds to set the bottom slightly.

4. Using a spatula, gently push the eggs from the edge of the pan towards the center, tilting the pan to allow the uncooked egg to flow to the edges.

5. When the eggs are mostly set but still a bit wet on top, add your desired meat filling(s) to one half of the omelette.

6. Use the spatula to fold the unfilled half of the omelette over the filled half.

7. Slide the omelette onto a plate and season with salt and pepper.

8. Optionally, you can top with a sprinkle of grated cheese.

9. Serve the omelette immediately while hot.

Repeat the process to make additional omelettes. Adjust the fillings to your preference. Enjoy your hearty carnivore•friendly omelette!

# 66. Beef bone broth

## Ingredient:

- 3•4 lbs beef bones (such as marrow bones, knuckle bones, oxtail)
- 1 onion, roughly chopped
- 2 carrots, roughly chopped
- 2 celery stalks, roughly chopped
- 2 tbsp apple cider vinegar
- 1 tsp salt
- Filtered water

## Instructions:

1. Preheat your oven to 400°F (200°C).

2. Spread the beef bones out on a large baking sheet and roast for 30•45 minutes, until browned.

3. Transfer the roasted bones to a large stockpot or slow cooker. Add the chopped onion, carrots, and celery.

4. Pour in enough filtered water to cover the bones and vegetables by 1•2 inches.

5. Stir in the apple cider vinegar. This helps extract the nutrients from the bones.

6. Bring the mixture to a boil over high heat. Once boiling, reduce heat to low, cover, and simmer for 24•48 hours, skimming any foam or fat that rises to the top.

7. After simmering, strain the broth through a fine mesh sieve, discarding the solids.

8. Season the broth with salt to taste.

9. Allow the broth to cool completely, then transfer to airtight containers and refrigerate for up to 1 week or freeze for up to 6 months.

Tips:
- Use a combination of beef bones like marrow bones, knuckle bones, and oxtail for maximum gelatin and nutrients.
- Roasting the bones first enhances the flavor.
- Add any other carnivore•friendly vegetables like garlic or ginger.
- Drink the broth on its own or use it as a base for soups and stews.

# 67. Chicken bone broth

## Ingredient:

- 3•4 lbs chicken bones (such as backs, necks, feet)
- 1 onion, roughly chopped
- 2 carrots, roughly chopped
- 2 celery stalks, roughly chopped
- 2 tbsp apple cider vinegar
- 1 tsp salt
- Filtered water

## Instructions:

1. Place the chicken bones in a large stockpot or slow cooker. Add the chopped onion, carrots, and celery.

2. Pour in enough filtered water to cover the bones and vegetables by 1•2 inches.

3. Stir in the apple cider vinegar. This helps extract the nutrients from the bones.

4. Bring the mixture to a boil over high heat. Once boiling, reduce heat to low, cover, and simmer for 12•24 hours, skimming any foam or fat that rises to the top.

5. After simmering, strain the broth through a fine mesh sieve, discarding the solids.

6. Season the broth with salt to taste.

7. Allow the broth to cool completely, then transfer to airtight containers and refrigerate for up to 1 week or freeze for up to 6 months.

Tips:
- Use a combination of chicken bones, feet, and necks for maximum gelatin and nutrients.

- Roast the bones first for deeper flavor.

- Add any other carnivore•friendly vegetables like garlic or ginger.

- Drink the broth on its own or use it as a base for soups and stews.

This nourishing chicken bone broth is perfect for a carnivore diet, providing collagen, protein, and minerals.

# 68. Lamb broth

**Ingredient:**

- 3 lbs lamb bones (marrow bones, knuckles, etc.)
- 1 onion, chopped
- 3 cloves garlic, minced
- 1 tbsp apple cider vinegar
- 1 tsp sea salt
- 1/2 tsp black pepper
- Water to cover

**Instructions:**

1. Place the lamb bones in a large stock pot and cover with water. Add the onion, garlic, apple cider vinegar, salt, and pepper.

2. Bring the pot to a boil, then reduce heat and let simmer for 8•12 hours, skimming any foam or fat that rises to the top. The longer it simmers, the more nutrients will be extracted from the bones.

3. Strain the broth through a fine mesh sieve, discarding the solids.

4. Allow the broth to cool, then skim off any solidified fat on the surface.

5. Store the broth in the refrigerator for up to 1 week or freeze for longer term storage.

This nutrient•dense lamb bone broth provides collagen, gelatin, minerals, and healthy fats that are beneficial for women following a carnivore diet. Enjoy the broth on its own or use it as a base for other dishes.

# 69. Beef stew

## Ingredient:

- 2 lbs beef chuck roast, cut into 1•inch cubes
- 1 cup beef bone broth
- 1 tbsp apple cider vinegar
- 1 tsp sea salt
- 1/2 tsp black pepper
- 1/2 tsp garlic powder
- 1/2 tsp onion powder
- 2 tbsp tallow or beef fat for cooking

## Instructions:

1. In a large pot or dutch oven, heat the tallow or beef fat over medium•high heat. Add the beef cubes and brown on all sides, about 3•5 minutes per side.

2. Once the beef is browned, add the beef bone broth, apple cider vinegar, salt, pepper, garlic powder, and onion powder. Stir to combine.

3. Bring the stew to a boil, then reduce heat to low, cover, and let simmer for 2•3 hours, until the beef is very tender.

4. Taste and adjust seasoning as needed.

5. Serve the beef stew warm. This dish is delicious on its own or can be served over cauliflower rice.

The long simmering time helps break down the connective tissue in the beef chuck, making it very tender. The bone broth provides collagen and minerals, while the apple cider vinegar aids digestion. This hearty stew is perfect for women following a carnivore diet.

# 70. Chicken soup

## Ingredient:

• 4 lbs chicken bones (backs, necks, feet)
• 1 whole chicken (3•4 lbs)
• 1 onion, chopped
• 3 cloves garlic, minced
• 1 tbsp apple cider vinegar
• 1 tsp sea salt
• 1/2 tsp black pepper
• Water to cover

## Instructions:

1. Place the chicken bones in a large stock pot and cover with water. Bring to a boil, then reduce heat and let simmer for 6•8 hours, skimming any foam or fat that rises to the top.

2. Add the whole chicken to the pot and continue simmering for another 2•3 hours, until the chicken is very tender and falling off the bone.

3. Remove the chicken from the pot and let cool slightly. Shred or chop the meat, discarding the skin and bones.

4. Add the chopped onion and garlic to the broth and continue simmering for 30 minutes.

5. Season the broth with the apple cider vinegar, salt, and pepper.

6. Add the shredded chicken back to the broth and heat through.

7. Serve the chicken soup warm. Can be stored in the refrigerator for up to 1 week or frozen for longer term storage.

This nutrient•dense chicken soup provides collagen, gelatin, and essential amino acids that are beneficial for women following a carnivore diet. The apple cider vinegar aids digestion.

# 71. Beef marrow soup

## Ingredient:

• 2 lbs beef marrow bones, cut into 1•inch pieces
• 1 onion, diced
• 3 cloves garlic, minced
• 1 tbsp apple cider vinegar
• 1 tsp sea salt
• 1/2 tsp black pepper
• 4 cups beef bone broth
• 2 tbsp tallow or beef fat for cooking

## Instructions:

1. In a large pot or dutch oven, heat the tallow or beef fat over medium•high heat. Add the beef marrow bones and brown on all sides, about 3•5 minutes per side.

2. Remove the browned marrow bones from the pot and set aside. Add the diced onion to the pot and sauté for 2•3 minutes until translucent.

3. Add the minced garlic and sauté for 1 minute until fragrant.

4. Pour in the beef bone broth and add the browned marrow bones back to the pot. Stir in the apple cider vinegar, salt, and pepper.

5. Bring the soup to a boil, then reduce heat to low, cover, and let simmer for 2•3 hours, until the marrow is very soft and falling out of the bones.

6. Using a slotted spoon, remove the marrow bones from the soup. Use a fork to scoop out the soft marrow and add it back to the broth.

7. Taste the soup and adjust seasoning as needed.

8. Serve the beef marrow soup warm. Can be stored in the refrigerator for up to 1 week or frozen for longer term storage.

This nourishing soup is rich in collagen, gelatin, and healthy fats from the beef marrow, making it an excellent choice for women following a carnivore diet. The apple cider vinegar aids digestion.

# 72. Steak salad (without dressings)

## Ingredient:

- 1 lb flank steak or ribeye steak
- 4 cups mixed greens (spinach, arugula, kale, etc.)
- 1/2 red onion, thinly sliced
- 1 avocado, sliced
- 2 hard boiled eggs, sliced
- Sea salt and black pepper to taste

## Instructions:

1. Season the steak generously with sea salt and black pepper.

2. Heat a cast iron skillet or grill pan over high heat. Cook the steak for 3•5 minutes per side, depending on thickness, until it reaches your desired doneness.

3. Remove the steak from the heat and let it rest for 5•10 minutes. Slice the steak against the grain into thin strips.

4. In a large salad bowl, combine the mixed greens, sliced red onion, avocado slices, and hard boiled egg slices.

5. Top the salad with the sliced steak.

6. Serve the steak salad as is, without any dressings. The natural juices from the steak will provide enough moisture and flavor.

This simple steak salad is packed with protein, healthy fats, and essential nutrients that are beneficial for women following a carnivore diet. The combination of greens, avocado, eggs, and steak creates a satisfying and nutrient•dense meal.

# 73. Chicken salad (without dressings)

## Ingredient:

• 2 lbs boneless, skinless chicken thighs
• 1 cup diced celery
• 1/2 cup diced red onion
• 2 hard boiled eggs, chopped
• 1 avocado, diced
• Sea salt and black pepper to taste

## Instructions:

1. Place the chicken thighs in a large pot and cover with water. Bring to a boil, then reduce heat and simmer for 20•25 minutes, until the chicken is cooked through.

2. Remove the chicken from the pot and let cool slightly. Shred or chop the chicken into bite•sized pieces.

3. In a large bowl, combine the shredded chicken, diced celery, diced red onion, chopped hard boiled eggs, and diced avocado.

4. Season the chicken salad with sea salt and black pepper to taste.

5. Serve the chicken salad as is, without any dressings. The natural juices from the chicken and avocado will provide enough moisture and flavor.

This simple chicken salad is a great option for women following a carnivore diet. It's packed with protein, healthy fats, and essential nutrients. The combination of chicken, vegetables, and eggs creates a satisfying and nutrient•dense meal.

# 74. Beef jerky (sugar•free)

## Ingredient:

• 2 lbs lean beef (such as flank steak or top round), sliced into thin strips
• 2 tsp sea salt
• 1 tsp black pepper
• 1 tsp garlic powder
• 1 tsp onion powder
• 1/2 tsp cayenne pepper (optional, for a spicy version)

## Instructions:

1. In a large bowl, combine the beef strips with the sea salt, black pepper, garlic powder, onion powder, and cayenne pepper (if using). Mix well to evenly coat the beef.

2. Arrange the seasoned beef strips in a single layer on dehydrator trays or baking sheets lined with parchment paper.

3. Dehydrate the beef jerky at 155°F for 6•8 hours, or until the jerky is dry and leathery, but still pliable. Flip the strips halfway through the drying process.

4. Alternatively, you can bake the jerky in the oven. Preheat the oven to 175°F and bake the jerky for 4•6 hours, flipping the strips occasionally, until fully dried.

5. Allow the beef jerky to cool completely before storing.

6. Store the jerky in an airtight container at room temperature for up to 2 weeks, or in the refrigerator for up to 1 month.

This sugar•free beef jerky is a great high•protein, low•carb snack option for women following a carnivore diet. The combination of spices provides flavor without added sugars.

# 75. Pork rinds

## Ingredient:

• Pork skin, with fat attached (about 1 lb)
• Sea salt

## Instructions:

1. Preheat your oven to 400°F (200°C).

2. Rinse the pork skin under cold water and pat it dry thoroughly with paper towels. Use a sharp knife to cut the skin into 1•inch wide strips.

3. Arrange the pork skin strips in a single layer on a baking sheet lined with parchment paper. Make sure the pieces are not touching each other.

4. Sprinkle the pork skin generously with sea salt.

5. Bake for 30•40 minutes, flipping the pieces halfway, until the pork rinds are puffed up and golden brown.

6. Remove the pork rinds from the oven and let them cool completely. They will continue to crisp up as they cool.

7. Once cooled, store the pork rinds in an airtight container at room temperature for up to 1 week.

Pork rinds are a great crunchy, high•protein snack option for women following a carnivore diet. The simple preparation allows the natural flavors of the pork to shine. Enjoy the pork rinds on their own or use them as a crunchy topping for other dishes.

# 76. Chicken wings (plain)

## Ingredient:

- 2 lbs chicken wings, drumettes and flats separated
- 1 tsp sea salt
- 1/2 tsp black pepper

## Instructions:

1. Preheat your oven to 400°F (200°C). Line a baking sheet with parchment paper.

2. Pat the chicken wings dry with paper towels and place them in a single layer on the prepared baking sheet.

3. Sprinkle the chicken wings evenly with the sea salt and black pepper, making sure to season both sides.

4. Bake the chicken wings for 40•45 minutes, flipping them halfway through, until they are crispy and cooked through.

5. Optionally, you can broil the wings for the last 2•3 minutes to get them extra crispy.

6. Serve the plain chicken wings warm. They can be enjoyed on their own or with a side of your favorite carnivore•friendly dipping sauce (such as melted butter or ranch dressing).

These simple, seasoned chicken wings are a great high•protein, low•carb option for women following a carnivore diet. The lack of breading or sugary sauces keeps the dish in line with the diet's principles. Enjoy these wings as a snack or as part of a larger carnivore•friendly meal.

# 77. Beef sticks

## Ingredient:

• 2 lbs lean ground beef
• 2 tsp sea salt
• 1 tsp black pepper
• 1 tsp garlic powder
• 1 tsp onion powder
• 1/2 tsp smoked paprika (optional)

## Instructions:

1. In a large bowl, combine the ground beef, sea salt, black pepper, garlic powder, onion powder, and smoked paprika (if using). Mix well until the seasonings are evenly distributed.

2. Divide the seasoned ground beef into 8 equal portions. Roll each portion into a long, thin stick shape, about 6•8 inches long.

3. Place the beef sticks on a parchment•lined baking sheet or dehydrator trays, making sure they are not touching each other.

4. Dehydrate the beef sticks at 155°F for 6•8 hours, or until they are dry and jerky•like in texture, but still pliable. Flip the sticks halfway through the drying process.

5. Alternatively, you can bake the beef sticks in the oven. Preheat the oven to 175°F and bake for 4•6 hours, flipping the sticks occasionally, until fully dried.

6. Allow the beef sticks to cool completely before storing.

7. Store the beef sticks in an airtight container at room temperature for up to 2 weeks, or in the refrigerator for up to 1 month.

These homemade beef sticks are a great high•protein, low•carb snack option for women following a carnivore diet. The simple seasoning allows the natural flavor of the beef to shine through.

# 78. Butter

## Ingredient:

• Heavy cream (preferably from grass•fed cows)

## Instructions:

1. Pour the heavy cream into a food processor or high•powered blender.

2. Process the cream on high speed for 5•10 minutes, until the cream separates into butter solids and buttermilk.

3. Once the butter has formed, stop the food processor and pour the contents through a fine mesh strainer or cheesecloth to separate the butter from the buttermilk.

4. Rinse the butter under cold running water, kneading it with your hands, to remove any remaining buttermilk. This will help the butter keep longer.

5. Shape the butter into a log or pat and place it on a piece of parchment paper or wax paper. Wrap it tightly and refrigerate until firm, about 30 minutes.

6. The butter can be stored in the refrigerator for up to 2 weeks or frozen for longer term storage.

This homemade butter is a great source of healthy fats and is perfect for women following a carnivore diet. It can be used for cooking, baking, or enjoyed on its own as a spread. The grass•fed cream provides additional nutrients and a rich, creamy flavor.

# 79. Ghee

**Ingredient:**

• 1 lb unsalted butter (preferably from grass•fed cows)

**Instructions:**

1. In a heavy•bottomed saucepan or pot, melt the butter over medium heat.

2. Once the butter has melted, reduce the heat to low and let the butter simmer gently. As it simmers, the butter will begin to foam and bubble.

3. Continue simmering the butter, stirring occasionally, for 20•30 minutes. You'll notice the butter will go through several stages:
    • First, it will foam and bubble.
    • Then, the foam will subside and small white milk solids will begin to form at the bottom of the pan.
    • Finally, the milk solids will turn golden brown, and the butter will become clear and fragrant.

4. Once the milk solids have turned golden brown, remove the pan from the heat. Carefully pour the clarified butter through a fine mesh strainer or cheesecloth to remove any remaining milk solids.

5. Allow the ghee to cool slightly, then transfer it to a clean, airtight container.

6. The ghee can be stored at room temperature for up to 6 months. It has a higher smoke point than regular butter, making it ideal for high•heat cooking.

Ghee is a great source of healthy fats and is perfect for women following a carnivore diet. It's lactose•free and has a rich, nutty flavor that can enhance the taste of many dishes.

# 80. Lard

**Ingredient:**

• Pork fat (leaf lard or fatback)

**Instructions:**

1. Gather the pork fat. You can use leaf lard (the fat around the kidneys) or fatback (the thick layer of fat on the back of the pig). Trim off any meat or skin attached to the fat.

2. Cut the pork fat into 1•inch cubes.

3. Place the cubed fat in a heavy•bottomed pot or Dutch oven. Add just enough water to cover the bottom of the pot, about 1/4 cup.

4. Heat the pot over medium•low heat, stirring occasionally, until the fat begins to render and melt, about 30•45 minutes.

5. Once the fat has fully melted, increase the heat to medium•high and continue cooking, stirring frequently, until the remaining pork cracklings (also called "cracklins") have turned golden brown, about 30•45 minutes more.

6. Carefully strain the hot lard through a fine mesh strainer or cheesecloth to remove any impurities or cracklings.

7. Allow the lard to cool slightly, then transfer it to clean, airtight containers. The lard can be stored at room temperature for up to 6 months.

8. The leftover cracklings can be reserved and used as a crunchy topping for dishes or enjoyed as a snack.

Lard is an excellent source of healthy fats and is perfect for women following a carnivore diet. It has a high smoke point, making it ideal for high•heat cooking and frying.

# 81. Tallow

## Ingredient:

• Beef fat (suet or leaf fat)

## Instructions:

1. Gather the beef fat. You can use suet (the hard fat around the kidneys and loins) or leaf fat (the fat around the internal organs). Trim off any meat or connective tissue attached to the fat.

2. Cut the beef fat into 1•inch cubes.

3. Place the cubed fat in a heavy•bottomed pot or Dutch oven. Add just enough water to cover the bottom of the pot, about 1/4 cup.

4. Heat the pot over medium•low heat, stirring occasionally, until the fat begins to render and melt, about 30•45 minutes.

5. Once the fat has fully melted, increase the heat to medium•high and continue cooking, stirring frequently, until the remaining beef cracklings have turned golden brown, about 30•45 minutes more.

6. Carefully strain the hot tallow through a fine mesh strainer or cheesecloth to remove any impurities or cracklings.

7. Allow the tallow to cool slightly, then transfer it to clean, airtight containers. The tallow can be stored at room temperature for up to 6 months.

8. The leftover cracklings can be reserved and used as a crunchy topping for dishes or enjoyed as a snack.

Tallow is an excellent source of healthy fats and is perfect for women following a carnivore diet. It has a high smoke point, making it ideal for high•heat cooking and frying.

# 82. Ground beef scramble

## Ingredient:

- 1 lb ground beef
- 1 onion, diced
- 2 cloves garlic, minced
- 1 bell pepper, chopped
- 4 eggs, beaten
- Salt and pepper to taste
- Optional: shredded cheese, hot sauce

## Instructions:

1. Brown the ground beef in a large skillet over medium heat.

2. Add onion, garlic, and bell pepper. Cook until vegetables are soft.

3. Pour in beaten eggs, stirring to combine.

4. Cook until eggs are set, stirring occasionally.

5. Season with salt and pepper.

6. Serve hot, topped with cheese or hot sauce if desired.

# 83. Herbal tea (non•sweetened)

## Ingredient:

• 1•2 tsp dried herbal tea blend (such as chamomile, peppermint, lemon balm, etc.)
• 8 oz hot water (just off the boil)

## Instructions:

1. Bring fresh, cold water to a boil in a kettle or on the stove.

2. Place the dried herbal tea blend in a teapot, mug, or infuser.

3. Pour the hot water over the herbs and let steep for 5•7 minutes.

4. Strain the tea leaves or remove the infuser, and enjoy your hot, unsweetened herbal tea.

Tips:
• Experiment with different herbal tea blends to find your favorite flavors.

• You can steep the tea for longer to extract more flavor, but be careful not to over•steep which can make the tea taste bitter.

• Avoid adding any sweeteners, milk, or other additives to keep this tea completely unsweetened.

• Drink the tea hot or let it cool slightly before enjoying.

# 84. Grilled meats

## Ingredient:

• 1•2 lbs of your choice of meat (e.g. chicken breasts, steak, pork chops, etc.)
• Olive oil or vegetable oil
• Salt and pepper
• Optional seasonings (e.g. garlic powder, onion powder, paprika, etc.)

## Instructions:

1. Prepare the grill for direct, high•heat cooking. Preheat the grill to medium•high heat (around 400•450°F).

2. Pat the meat dry with paper towels and brush or drizzle with a light coating of oil. Season generously with salt, pepper, and any other desired seasonings.

3. Place the seasoned meat directly on the preheated grill grates. Cover the grill and cook for 4•6 minutes per side, depending on the thickness of the meat, until it reaches your desired doneness.

- For chicken, cook until the internal temperature reaches 165°F.
- For steak, cook to your preferred doneness (e.g. medium•rare, medium, medium•well).
- For pork, cook until the internal temperature reaches 145°F.

4. Use tongs or a spatula to flip the meat, being careful not to pierce it with a fork, which can cause the juices to escape.

5. Once the meat is cooked to your liking, transfer it to a clean cutting board or plate. Let it rest for 5•10 minutes before slicing or serving.

Tips:
• Allow the meat to come to room temperature before grilling for more even cooking.

• Baste the meat with a bit of oil or marinade during cooking for extra flavor.

• Adjust the grill temperature as needed to prevent burning.

• Experiment with different seasonings and marinades to find your favorite flavors.

Enjoy your perfectly grilled meats!

# 85. Roasted meats

## Ingredient:

• 2•3 lbs of your choice of meat (e.g. beef roast, pork loin, chicken, etc.)
• Olive oil or vegetable oil
• Salt and pepper
• Optional seasonings (e.g. garlic powder, onion powder, dried herbs, etc.)

## Instructions:

1. Preheat your oven to 375°F (190°C).

2. Pat the meat dry with paper towels and rub it all over with a light coating of oil. Season generously with salt, pepper, and any other desired seasonings.

3. Place the seasoned meat in a roasting pan or baking dish. If roasting a larger cut of meat, you can optionally place it on a wire rack set inside the roasting pan to allow the fat to drip away.

**4. Roast the meat in the preheated oven, uncovered, until it reaches your desired doneness:**

  • For beef, roast to an internal temperature of 125•130°F for medium•rare, 135•140°F for medium, or 145•150°F for medium•well.
  • For pork, roast to an internal temperature of 145°F.
  • For chicken, roast to an internal temperature of 165°F.

  **The cooking time will vary depending on the size and cut of the meat, but as a general guideline:**
  • Beef roast: 15•20 minutes per pound
  • Pork loin: 20•25 minutes per pound
  • Whole chicken: 60•90 minutes

5. Once the meat has reached the desired doneness, remove it from the oven and let it rest for 10•15 minutes before slicing or serving. This allows the juices to redistribute throughout the meat.

Tips:
• Use a meat thermometer to ensure the meat is cooked to your preferred doneness.
• Baste the meat with the pan juices during roasting for extra flavor and moisture.
• For crispier skin on poultry, pat the skin dry and rub it with a bit of oil before seasoning.
• Experiment with different seasoning blends to find your favorite flavors.

# 86. Pan-seared meats

## Ingredient:

• 1•2 lbs of your choice of meat (e.g. steak, pork chops, chicken breasts)
• Olive oil or vegetable oil
• Salt and pepper
• Optional seasonings (e.g. garlic powder, onion powder, dried herbs)

## Instructions:

1. Pat the meat dry with paper towels and season it generously with salt, pepper, and any other desired seasonings.

2. Heat a large, heavy•bottomed skillet (such as cast iron) over high heat. Add just enough oil to lightly coat the bottom of the pan.

3. When the oil is shimmering hot, carefully add the seasoned meat to the pan. Make sure not to overcrowd the pan, as this can cause the meat to steam rather than sear.

4. Sear the meat for 3•5 minutes per side, depending on the thickness, until a nice brown crust forms. Avoid moving the meat too much during this time to allow for proper searing.

5. Flip the meat and continue cooking for another 3•5 minutes, or until it reaches your desired doneness:

   • For steak, aim for an internal temperature of 125•130°F for medium•rare, 135•140°F for medium, or 145•150°F for medium•well.
   • For pork chops, cook to an internal temperature of 145°F.
   • For chicken breasts, cook to an internal temperature of 165°F.

6. Once the meat is cooked to your liking, transfer it to a clean cutting board or plate. Let it rest for 5•10 minutes before slicing or serving.

Tips:
• Pat the meat very dry before seasoning to ensure a good sear.
• Use a heavy, oven•safe skillet to get a nice, even sear.
• Avoid overcrowding the pan, as this can cause the meat to steam rather than sear.
• Baste the meat with the hot oil or pan juices during cooking for extra flavor.
• Let the meat rest before slicing to allow the juices to redistribute.
• Experiment with different seasoning blends to find your favorite flavors

# 87. Sous-vide meats

**Ingredient:**

• 1•2 lbs of your choice of meat (e.g. steak, pork chops, chicken breasts)
• Salt and pepper
• Optional seasonings (e.g. garlic powder, onion powder, dried herbs)
• Butter or oil (for searing, if desired)

***Equipment Needed:***
• Sous•vide water bath or immersion circulator
• Resealable plastic bags or vacuum•sealed bags

**Instructions:**

1. Season the meat generously with salt, pepper, and any other desired seasonings.

2. Place the seasoned meat in a resealable plastic bag or vacuum•sealed bag, making sure to remove as much air as possible.

3. Set up your sous•vide water bath or immersion circulator to the desired temperature:
   • For steak, 130•135°F for medium•rare, 140•145°F for medium
   • For pork, 145°F
   • For chicken, 165°F

4. Carefully lower the bagged meat into the water bath, making sure it is fully submerged. If using a resealable bag, you may need to weigh it down with a clip or spoon to keep it submerged.

5. Cook the meat in the water bath for the following times:
   • Steak: 1•4 hours, depending on thickness
   • Pork: 1•4 hours, depending on thickness
   • Chicken: 1•4 hours, depending on thickness

6. Once the meat has finished cooking, remove it from the water bath. If you want a seared crust, pat the meat dry and sear it in a hot pan with a bit of butter or oil for 1•2 minutes per side.

7. Let the meat rest for 5•10 minutes before slicing and serving.

Enjoy your perfectly cooked, tender, and flavorful sous•vide meats!

# 88. Slow-cooked meats

## Ingredient:

• 2•3 lbs of your choice of meat (e.g. beef chuck roast, pork shoulder, chicken thighs)
• Olive oil or vegetable oil
• Salt and pepper
• Optional seasonings (e.g. garlic powder, onion powder, dried herbs, spices)
• Broth or liquid (e.g. beef/chicken stock, wine, tomato sauce)

### *Equipment Needed:*
• Slow cooker or crockpot

## Instructions:

1. Season the meat generously with salt, pepper, and any other desired seasonings.

2. Heat a large skillet over medium•high heat and add a small amount of oil. Sear the meat on all sides until a nice brown crust forms, about 2•3 minutes per side. This step is optional but helps develop more flavor.

3. Transfer the seared meat to a slow cooker. If you didn't sear the meat, simply place the seasoned meat in the slow cooker.

4. Add enough broth, wine, or other liquid to the slow cooker to come about halfway up the sides of the meat. You can also add vegetables, such as onions, carrots, and potatoes, if desired.

5. Cover the slow cooker and cook the meat on low for 8•10 hours or on high for 4•6 hours, until the meat is very tender and easily shreds or pulls apart.

6. Once the meat is cooked, remove it from the slow cooker and shred or slice it, as desired. You can also leave the meat whole and serve it in the cooking liquid.

7. Taste the cooking liquid and adjust the seasoning if needed. You can thicken the liquid into a sauce by simmering it on the stovetop or mixing in a cornstarch slurry.

8. Serve the slow•cooked meat with the cooking liquid/sauce and your choice of sides, such as mashed potatoes, rice, or roasted vegetables.

Enjoy your delicious, fall•off•the•bone slow•cooked meats!

# 89. Smoked meats

## Ingredient:

• 2•3 lbs of your choice of meat (e.g. brisket, pork shoulder, chicken)
• Olive oil or vegetable oil
• Dry rub seasoning (e.g. salt, pepper, paprika, garlic powder, brown sugar)

### *Equipment Needed:*
• Smoker or grill with a smoking box/tray
• Wood chips or pellets (e.g. hickory, mesquite, apple)

## Instructions:
1. Prepare the meat:
   • Pat the meat dry with paper towels.
   • Rub the meat all over with a thin layer of oil.
   • Apply a generous amount of your desired dry rub seasoning, massaging it into the meat.
   • Let the seasoned meat sit at room temperature for 30 minutes to 1 hour before smoking.

2. Prepare the smoker or grill:
   • If using a smoker, follow the manufacturer's instructions to get it preheated to 225•250°F.
   • If using a grill, set up for indirect heat and place a smoking box or tray filled with wood chips/pellets over the heat source.

3. Smoke the meat:
   • Place the seasoned meat in the smoker or on the grill grates, making sure it's not directly over the heat source.
   • Add the wood chips or pellets to the smoking box/tray, if using a grill.
   • Close the lid and smoke the meat, maintaining the temperature between 225•250°F, for the following approximate times:
   • Brisket: 8•12 hours
   • Pork shoulder: 8•12 hours
   • Chicken: 2•4 hours
   • Replenish the wood chips/pellets as needed to maintain a steady smoke.
   • Use a meat thermometer to monitor the internal temperature of the meat.

4. Finish and rest the meat:
   • Once the meat reaches the desired internal temperature (brisket: 195•205°F, pork: 195•205°F, chicken: 165°F), remove it from the smoker or grill.
   • Let the meat rest for 30 minutes to 1 hour before slicing or pulling.

# 90. Bacon and eggs

**Ingredient:**

- 4•6 slices of bacon
- 2•4 eggs
- Salt and pepper to taste

**Instructions:**

1. Place bacon in a cold skillet. Cook over medium heat, turning occasionally, until crisp (about 8•10 minutes).

2. Remove bacon, drain on paper towels. Leave about 1 tablespoon of bacon fat in the pan.

3. Crack eggs into the skillet with bacon fat.

4. Cook sunny•side up, or flip for over•easy. About 3•4 minutes total.

5. Season eggs with salt and pepper.

6. Serve eggs with bacon on the side.

# 91. Korean BBQ (meat only)

## Ingredient:

- 1 lb beef sirloin or flank steak, thinly sliced against the grain
- 1/2 cup soy sauce
- 1/4 cup brown sugar
- 3 cloves garlic, minced
- 2 tbsp sesame oil
- 1 tbsp rice vinegar
- 1 tsp grated ginger
- 1/2 tsp black pepper
- Sesame seeds for garnish
- Lettuce leaves, for serving
- Sautéed vegetables (such as spinach, bean sprouts, carrots), for serving

## Marinade:

1. In a large bowl, combine the soy sauce, brown sugar, garlic, sesame oil, rice vinegar, ginger, and black pepper. Add the sliced beef and toss to coat evenly. Cover and marinate in the refrigerator for at least 30 minutes, up to 4 hours.

## Cooking:

2. Heat a grill pan or outdoor grill to medium•high heat. Working in batches if needed, cook the marinated beef for 2•3 minutes per side until charred and cooked through.

3. Transfer the cooked beef to a serving platter and sprinkle with sesame seeds.

4. Serve the Korean BBQ with lettuce leaves, sautéed vegetables, and any desired sauces or condiments on the side. Encourage guests to wrap the beef in the lettuce leaves.

# 92. Brazilian churrasco

## Ingredient:

• 1 lb beef tenderloin, cut into 1•inch thick steaks
• 1 lb chicken thighs, bone•in and skin•on
• 1 lb pork loin chops, 1•inch thick
• 1 tbsp coarse sea salt
• 1 tsp ground black pepper
• 1 tsp garlic powder
• 1 tsp onion powder
• 1 tbsp olive oil

### *Chimichurri Sauce:*
• 1 cup fresh parsley, finely chopped
• 3 cloves garlic, minced
• 2 tbsp red wine vinegar
• 1/4 cup olive oil
• 1 tsp dried oregano
• 1/4 tsp red pepper flakes
• Salt and pepper to taste

## Instructions:

1. Prepare the meats: Pat the beef, chicken, and pork dry with paper towels. Season all over with the salt, pepper, garlic powder, and onion powder.

2. Make the chimichurri sauce: In a small bowl, combine the parsley, garlic, vinegar, olive oil, oregano, and red pepper flakes. Season with salt and pepper to taste. Set aside.

3. Preheat your grill or grill pan to high heat.

4. Brush the meats lightly with olive oil. Grill the beef for 3•5 minutes per side for medium•rare, the chicken for 6•8 minutes per side, and the pork for 4•6 minutes per side, until cooked through.

5. Transfer the grilled meats to a cutting board and let rest for 5 minutes.

6. Slice the beef and pork against the grain. Serve the meats warm, accompanied by the chimichurri sauce on the side.

This carnivore•friendly Brazilian churrasco is packed with protein and healthy fats, making it an excellent choice for women following a carnivore diet. Enjoy!

# 93. Argentine asado

## Ingredient:

• 2 lbs beef short ribs
• 2 lbs beef flank steak
• 2 lbs chorizo sausages
• 1 lb morcilla (blood sausage)
• 1 lb chicken thighs, bone•in and skin•on
• Coarse sea salt
• Freshly ground black pepper

### *Chimichurri Sauce:*
• 1 cup fresh parsley, finely chopped
• 3 cloves garlic, minced
• 1/2 cup olive oil
• 2 tbsp red wine vinegar
• 1 tsp dried oregano
• 1/4 tsp red pepper flakes
• Salt and pepper to taste

## Instructions:

1. Prepare the meats: Pat the beef, chorizo, morcilla, and chicken dry with paper towels. Season generously with coarse sea salt and black pepper.

2. Make the chimichurri sauce: In a small bowl, combine the parsley, garlic, olive oil, vinegar, oregano, and red pepper flakes. Season with salt and pepper to taste. Set aside.

3. Prepare your grill for direct, high•heat cooking. If using a charcoal grill, let the coals burn until they're covered with a light gray ash.

4. Grill the meats, working in batches if necessary, until cooked to your desired doneness:
   • Beef short ribs: 6•8 minutes per side
   • Beef flank steak: 4•6 minutes per side for medium•rare
   • Chorizo and morcilla sausages: 8•10 minutes, turning occasionally
   • Chicken thighs: 12•15 minutes per side

5. Transfer the grilled meats to a cutting board and let rest for 5•10 minutes. Slice the beef and sausages and arrange on a platter. Serve the asado with the chimichurri sauce on the side.

Enjoy this authentic Argentine asado experience! The combination of grilled meats and the vibrant chimichurri sauce is truly delicious.

# 94. Greek souvlaki (meat skewers)

## Ingredient:

• 1 lb boneless, skinless chicken thighs, cut into 1•inch cubes
• 1 lb beef tenderloin, cut into 1•inch cubes
• 1 lb pork loin, cut into 1•inch cubes
• 2 tbsp olive oil
• 2 tsp dried oregano
• 1 tsp garlic powder
• 1 tsp onion powder
• 1 tsp coarse sea salt
• 1/2 tsp ground black pepper

*Tzatziki Sauce:*
• 1 cup full•fat Greek yogurt
• 1 cucumber, grated and squeezed dry
• 2 cloves garlic, minced
• 1 tbsp fresh lemon juice
• 1 tsp dried dill
• Salt and pepper to taste

## Instructions:

1. In a large bowl, combine the cubed chicken, beef, and pork. Add the olive oil, oregano, garlic powder, onion powder, salt, and pepper. Toss to coat the meat evenly.

2. Thread the marinated meat onto metal or wooden skewers, leaving a small space between each piece.

3. Preheat your grill or grill pan to medium•high heat.

4. Grill the souvlaki skewers for 8•10 minutes, turning occasionally, until the meat is cooked through and lightly charred.

5. Make the tzatziki sauce: In a small bowl, mix together the Greek yogurt, grated cucumber, garlic, lemon juice, and dried dill. Season with salt and pepper to taste.

6. Serve the grilled souvlaki skewers warm, accompanied by the tzatziki sauce on the side.

This carnivore•friendly Greek souvlaki is a great source of protein and healthy fats, making it an excellent choice for women following a carnivore diet. Enjoy!

# 95. Japanese yakiniku

## Ingredient:

- 1 lb beef short ribs, thinly sliced
- 1 lb beef tongue, thinly sliced
- 1 lb beef sirloin, thinly sliced
- 1 lb chicken thighs, thinly sliced
- 2 tbsp sesame oil
- 2 tbsp soy sauce
- 1 tbsp mirin
- 1 tbsp rice vinegar
- 2 cloves garlic, minced
- 1 tsp grated ginger
- 1/2 tsp ground black pepper

***Dipping Sauces:***
- Ponzu sauce (equal parts soy sauce and citrus juice)
- Grated daikon radish with soy sauce

## Instructions:

1. In a large bowl, combine the thinly sliced beef short ribs, beef tongue, beef sirloin, and chicken thighs.

2. In a small bowl, whisk together the sesame oil, soy sauce, mirin, rice vinegar, garlic, ginger, and black pepper. Pour the marinade over the meat and toss to coat evenly. Cover and refrigerate for at least 30 minutes, up to 2 hours.

3. Preheat your grill or grill pan to high heat.

4. Working in batches if necessary, grill the marinated meat for 2·3 minutes per side, or until cooked to your desired doneness.

5. Serve the grilled yakiniku immediately, accompanied by the ponzu sauce and grated daikon radish with soy sauce for dipping.

This carnivore·friendly Japanese yakiniku is packed with protein and healthy fats, making it an excellent choice for women following a carnivore diet. The thin slices of meat cook quickly, and the flavorful dipping sauces add a delicious touch. Enjoy!

# 96. Mongolian BBQ

## Ingredient:

• 1 lb beef sirloin, thinly sliced
• 1 lb lamb loin, thinly sliced
• 1 lb chicken thighs, thinly sliced
• 2 tbsp sesame oil
• 2 tbsp soy sauce
• 1 tbsp rice vinegar
• 1 tbsp grated ginger
• 2 cloves garlic, minced
• 1 tsp ground black pepper
• 1/2 tsp red pepper flakes (optional)

***Toppings***:
• Thinly sliced green onions
• Toasted sesame seeds
• Grated daikon radish

**Instructions**:
1. In a large bowl, combine the thinly sliced beef, lamb, and chicken.

2. In a small bowl, whisk together the sesame oil, soy sauce, rice vinegar, grated ginger, minced garlic, black pepper, and red pepper flakes (if using).

3. Pour the marinade over the meat and toss to coat evenly. Cover and refrigerate for at least 30 minutes, up to 2 hours.

4. Heat a large, flat•bottomed pan or griddle over high heat. Working in batches if necessary, cook the marinated meat for 2•3 minutes per side, or until cooked through and lightly charred.

5. Transfer the cooked meat to a serving platter and top with the sliced green onions, toasted sesame seeds, and grated daikon radish.

6. Serve the Mongolian BBQ immediately, allowing your guests to assemble their own bowls.

This carnivore•friendly Mongolian BBQ is a great source of protein and healthy fats, making it an excellent choice for women following a carnivore diet. The thin slices of meat cook quickly, and the flavorful toppings add a delicious touch. Enjoy!

# 97. Turkish kebabs

## Ingredient:

- 1 lb ground lamb
- 1 lb ground beef
- 2 tbsp olive oil
- 2 tsp ground cumin
- 1 tsp paprika
- 1 tsp garlic powder
- 1 tsp onion powder
- 1 tsp dried oregano
- 1 tsp coarse sea salt
- 1/2 tsp ground black pepper

### *Yogurt Sauce:*

- 1 cup full•fat Greek yogurt
- 1 tbsp lemon juice
- 1 clove garlic, minced
- 1 tsp dried dill
- Salt and pepper to taste

## Instructions:

1. In a large bowl, combine the ground lamb, ground beef, olive oil, cumin, paprika, garlic powder, onion powder, oregano, salt, and pepper. Mix well until the spices are evenly distributed.

2. Divide the meat mixture into 8 equal portions and shape each one into a long, thin kebab shape, about 6 inches long and 1 inch wide.

3. Preheat your grill or grill pan to medium•high heat.

4. Grill the kebabs for 8•10 minutes, turning occasionally, until cooked through and lightly charred on the outside.

5. Make the yogurt sauce: In a small bowl, mix together the Greek yogurt, lemon juice, minced garlic, and dried dill. Season with salt and pepper to taste. Serve the grilled Turkish kebabs warm, accompanied by the yogurt sauce on the side.

This carnivore•friendly Turkish kebab recipe is a great source of protein and healthy fats, making it an excellent choice for women following a carnivore diet. The combination of ground lamb and beef, along with the flavorful spices, creates a delicious and satisfying meal.

# 98. Indian tandoori meats

## Ingredient:

- 1 tsp paprika
- 1 tsp ground cumin
- 1 tsp cayenne pepper
- 1 tsp coarse sea salt
- 1/2 tsp ground black pepper

*Garnishes:*
- Lemon wedges
- Chopped cilantro

- 1 lb boneless, skinless chicken thighs, cut into 1•inch cubes
- 1 lb lamb loin, cut into 1•inch cubes
- 1 lb beef tenderloin, cut into 1•inch cubes
- 1 cup full•fat Greek yogurt
- 2 tbsp lemon juice
- 2 tbsp grated ginger
- 4 cloves garlic, minced
- 2 tsp garam masala

## Instructions:

1. In a large bowl, combine the cubed chicken, lamb, and beef.

2. In a separate bowl, whisk together the Greek yogurt, lemon juice, grated ginger, minced garlic, garam masala, paprika, cumin, cayenne pepper, salt, and black pepper.

3. Pour the yogurt marinade over the meat and toss to coat evenly. Cover and refrigerate for at least 2 hours, up to 24 hours.

4. Preheat your oven to 400°F (200°C) or prepare your grill for high•heat cooking.

5. If using the oven, thread the marinated meat onto metal or wooden skewers. Place the skewers on a baking sheet and roast for 15•20 minutes, turning occasionally, until the meat is cooked through.

6. If grilling, thread the marinated meat onto skewers and grill for 8•10 minutes, turning occasionally, until the meat is cooked through.

7. Transfer the tandoori meats to a serving platter and garnish with lemon wedges and chopped cilantro.

Serve the Indian tandoori meats warm, with any desired low•carb accompaniments, such as a simple salad or steamed vegetables.

This carnivore•friendly tandoori dish is a great source of protein and healthy fats, making it an excellent choice for women following a carnivore diet. The yogurt marinade helps keep the meat tender and flavorful.

# 99. Sugar•free mousse

## Ingredient:

• 2 cups bone broth
• 2 tablespoons unflavored gelatin powder
• Optional: herbs, spices, or lemon juice for flavor

## Instructions:

1. Pour 1/2 cup of cold bone broth into a bowl. Sprinkle the gelatin over it and let it bloom for 5•10 minutes.

2. Heat the remaining 1 1/2 cups of bone broth until hot but not boiling.

3. Pour the hot broth into the bloomed gelatin mixture and stir until completely dissolved.

4. Add any optional flavorings if desired.

5. Pour the mixture into molds or a container.

6. Refrigerate for at least 4 hours or until set.

This recipe creates a savory, protein•rich gelatin. The texture will be firmer than commercial flavored gelatins due to the higher protein content of bone broth.

# 100. Sausage patties

## Ingredient:

- 1 lb ground pork (or a mix of pork and beef)
- 1 tsp salt
- 1 tsp dried sage
- 1/2 tsp ground black pepper
- 1/4 tsp dried thyme
- 1/4 tsp dried rosemary
- 1/4 tsp garlic powder
- 1/4 tsp onion powder
- Pinch of red pepper flakes (optional)
- 1 tbsp maple syrup or brown sugar (optional, for sweetness)

## Instructions:

1. Mix all ingredients in a bowl until well combined.

2. Form into 2•3 inch patties, about 1/2 inch thick.

3. Cook in a skillet over medium heat for about 4•5 minutes per side, until browned and cooked through.

This recipe is versatile • you can adjust the seasonings to your taste. Some variations include adding fennel seeds for an Italian flavor or using different types of meat.

# 101. Steak and eggs

## Ingredient:

• 1 steak (ribeye, sirloin, or your preferred cut)
• 2•4 eggs
• Salt and pepper
• Butter or oil for cooking
• Optional herbs (like parsley or chives) for garnish

## Instructions:

1. Season the steak with salt and pepper.

2. Heat a skillet over medium•high heat. Add a bit of oil or butter.

3. Cook the steak to your desired doneness:
   • Rare: 2•3 minutes per side
   • Medium: 3•4 minutes per side
   • Well•done: 4•5 minutes per side

4. Remove steak and let it rest.

5. In the same pan, lower heat to medium and cook eggs to your preference (sunny•side up, over•easy, scrambled, etc.).

6. Slice the steak against the grain.

7. Serve the steak with eggs on the side.

This dish is often accompanied by hash browns or toast. You can also add hollandaise sauce for a richer meal.

# 102. Breakfast steak

## Ingredient:

- Thin•cut steak (like minute steak, cube steak, or thin sirloin)
- Salt and pepper
- Butter or oil for cooking
- Optional seasonings: garlic powder, onion powder, or steak seasoning

## Instructions:

1. Season the steak with salt, pepper, and any additional seasonings.

2. Heat a skillet over medium•high heat. Add a small amount of butter or oil.

3. Cook the steak for about 2•3 minutes per side for medium doneness. Adjust time for thicker cuts or different preferences.

4. Let the steak rest for a few minutes before serving.

Breakfast steaks are often served with eggs, hash browns, or toast. They can also be used in breakfast sandwiches or burritos.

As we conclude ***100+ Recipes Carnivore Diet Cookbook for Men: Fuel Your Strength and Vitality with Delicious Meat-Based Recipes***, we hope this culinary journey has inspired you to embrace the power of the carnivore diet and its potential to enhance your strength, vitality, and overall well-being.

**Reflecting on Your Journey**

Throughout this cookbook, you've explored a diverse array of meat-based recipes designed to satisfy your palate while nourishing your body with essential nutrients. From hearty breakfasts to savory dinners and indulgent desserts, each dish has been crafted to support your goals of optimizing performance and maintaining robust health.

**Key Takeaways**

- ***Empowerment Through Nutrition:*** You've learned how the carnivore diet can provide the protein, vitamins, and minerals necessary to support muscle growth, recovery, and sustained energy levels throughout your day.

- ***Simplicity and Satisfaction:*** The recipes in this book have shown that eating well doesn't have to be complicated. With simple, flavorful dishes, you can enjoy delicious meals that fuel your body without unnecessary complexity.

- ***Holistic Health Approach:*** Beyond diet, this cookbook has emphasized the importance of holistic health practices such as regular exercise, adequate hydration, and effective stress management. These elements work in harmony with your dietary choices to promote overall vitality.

- ***Continual Growth and Exploration:*** Your journey with the carnivore diet is a dynamic process. Continue to explore new recipes, adapt your diet to meet your evolving needs, and celebrate the positive changes you experience along the way.

**Looking Ahead**

As you continue to incorporate the principles of the carnivore diet into your lifestyle, remember to listen to your body's signals and adjust accordingly. Share your experiences with others, seek support when needed, and revel in the newfound energy and vitality that come from fueling yourself with nutrient-dense, meat-based meals.

Thank you for allowing us to be a part of your journey towards better health and enhanced performance. May this cookbook continue to inspire you to discover the joys of cooking and eating delicious, meat-centric dishes that support your strength and vitality.